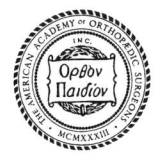

American Academy of Orthopaedic Surgeons
6300 North River Road
Rosemont, Illinois 60018
1-800-626-6726

D1808782

The Rotator Cuff

Current Concepts and Complex Problems

EDITED BY
JOSEPH P. IANNOTTI, MD, PhD

Professor, Orthopaedic Surgery
Chief, Shoulder and Elbow Service
University of Pennsylvania
Philadelphia, Pennsylvania

CONTRIBUTORS
Louis U. Bigliani, MD
Larry D. Field, MD
Evan L. Flatow, MD
Christian Gerber, MD
Charles W. Hartzog, MD

Joseph P. Iannotti, MD, PhD
Mark D. Miller, MD
Capt. R. John Naranja, Jr, MD
Felix H. Savoie, MD
Jonathan B. Ticker, MD
Jon J.P. Warner, MD

SERIES EDITOR
Thomas R. Johnson, MD

The American Academy of Orthopaedic Surgeons Monograph Series is dedicated to Wendy O. Schmidt, American Academy of Orthopaedic Surgeons senior medical editor, 1987-1991.

THE ROTATOR CUFF
American Academy of Orthopaedic Surgeons

The material presented in *The Rotator Cuff: Current Concepts and Complex Problems* has been made available by the American Academy of Orthopaedic Surgeons for educational purposes only. This material is not intended to present the only, or necessarily best, methods or procedures for the medical situations discussed, but rather is intended to represent an approach, view, statement, or opinion of the author(s) or producer(s), which may be helpful to others who face similar situations.

Some drugs or medical devices demonstrated in Academy education programs or materials have not been cleared by the Food and Drug Administration (FDA) or have been cleared by the FDA for specific uses only. The FDA has stated that it is the responsibility of the physician to determine the FDA clearance status of each drug or device he or she wishes to use in clinical practice.

Furthermore, any statements about commercial products are solely the opinion of the author(s) and do not represent an Academy endorsement or evaluation of these products. These statements may not be used in advertising or for any commercial purpose.

Library of Congress Cataloging-in-Publications Data
The Rotator Cuff: Current Concepts and Complex Problems
edited by Joseph P. Iannotti, MD, PhD

ISBN 0-89203-171-9

CONTENTS

CONTRIBUTORS

Louis U. Bigliani, MD
Chief, The Shoulder Service
New York Orthopaedic Hospital
Columbia-Presbyterian Medical Center
Professor of Orthopaedic Surgery
College of Physicians and Surgeons
Columbia University
New York, New York

Larry D. Field, MD
Co-Director, Upper Extremity Service
Mississippi Sportsmedicine
Jackson, Mississippi

Evan L. Flatow, MD
Associate Chief, The Shoulder Service
Professor of Orthopaedic Surgery
New York Orthopaedic Hospital
Columbia-Presbyterian Medical Center
College of Physicians and Surgeons
Columbia University
New York, New York

Christian Gerber, MD
Professor and Chairman
Department of Orthopaedic Surgery
University of Zürich
Zürich, Switzerland

Charles W. Hartzog, MD
Fellow in Sportsmedicine and Shoulder Surgery
Upper Extremity Service
Mississippi Sportsmedicine
Jackson, Mississippi

Joseph P. Iannotti, MD, PhD
Professor, Orthopaedic Surgery
Chief, Shoulder and Elbow Service
University of Pennsylvania
Philadelphia, Pennsylvania

Mark D. Miller, MD
The Shoulder Service
New York Orthopaedic Hospital
Columbia Presbyterian Medical Center
New York, New York

Capt. R. John Naranja, Jr, MD
Chief, Department of Orthopaedics
Minot Air Force Base, North Dakota
USAF Medical Corps
Minot Air Force Base, North Dakota

Felix H. Savoie, MD
Co-Director, Upper Extremity Service
Mississippi Sportsmedicine
Jackson, Mississippi

Jonathan B. Ticker, MD
Island Orthopaedics and Sports Medicine, PC
Massapequa, New York

Jon J.P. Warner, MD
Director, Shoulder Service
Associate Professor of Orthopaedic Surgery
University of Pittsburgh
Pittsburgh, Pennsylvania

PREFACE

Since the publication in 1991 of *Rotator Cuff Disorders,* the first monograph on the rotator cuff in the AAOS series, there have been several important advances in the understanding of the biology of cuff tissue and in the biomechanics and kinematics of the shoulder, rotator cuff, and cora-coacromial arch. More experience has been gained in arthroscopic techniques and the results thereof for the management of rotator cuff tears and acromioclavicular arthritis. In addition, bio-mechanical studies have advanced understanding of the preferred techniques for tendon to bone fix-ation. The management of the massive cuff tear has always challenged even the most experienced surgeon; advances in and a more thorough description of the techniques for tendon transfer and tendon repair are included in this monograph.

Finally, the diagnosis and management of compli-cations of rotator cuff surgery are more thoroughly described.

This monograph was developed to discuss these most recent advances in the management of rotator cuff tears and to supplement the material presented in the first monograph. I would like to acknowledge the superb effort and expertise of the contributing authors. Without their efforts, this monograph would not have been possible. I would also like to thank the staff of the AAOS Publications Department for their tireless efforts and expertise.

JOSEPH P. IANNOTTI, MD, PhD

BIOMECHANICS OF THE CORACOACROMIAL ARCH AND ROTATOR CUFF; KINEMATICS AND CONTACT OF THE SUBACROMIAL SPACE

MARK D. MILLER, MD, EVAN L. FLATOW, MD, LOUIS U. BIGLIANI, MD

INTRODUCTION

In the past two decades much new information has become available about rotator cuff disorders of the shoulder. Arthroscopic visualization of the undersurface (articular side) of the cuff tendons, arthroscopic inspection of the subacromial space, and magnetic resonance imaging of the rotator cuff tendons and muscles have opened new windows of understanding in rotator cuff disease. Anatomic, biochemical, biomechanical, and pathologic studies have similarly expanded the knowledge base of the various characteristics of cuff disorders. Surgical techniques, both open and arthroscopic, have evolved in parallel with these clinical and basic science investigations.

This section will review the anatomy, biomechanics, and kinematics of the coracoacromial arch, the subacromial space, and the rotator cuff. These areas will be discussed in the context of understanding the etiology of cuff disease, the pathomechanics of rotator cuff failure, and the rationale for therapeutic interventions.

ANATOMY

MUSCLE AND TENDON ANATOMY

There are 26 muscles controlling the shoulder girdle, four of which make up the rotator cuff. The subscapularis arises from the anterior surface of the scapula and inserts onto the lesser tuberosity of the proximal humerus. The upper two thirds of this muscle is innervated by the upper subscapular nerve (C5) and the lower one third is innervated by the lower subscapular nerve (C6). The origin of the supraspinatus is the supraspinatus fossa of the scapula, and its insertion is the upper aspect of the greater tuberosity after passing beneath the acromion and the acromioclavicular joint. It is innervated by the suprascapular nerve (C5 and C6 from the superior trunk of the brachial plexus), which passes inferior to the transverse scapular ligament with motor roots to the supraspinatus branching within 1 cm of the notch then coursing obliquely and laterally to the base of the scapular spine.[1] The infraspinatus arises from the infraspinatus fossa of the scapula and attaches to the posterolateral aspect of the greater tuberosity. The suprascapular nerve curves medially from the base of the scapular spine to innervate the supraspinatus muscle within 1 cm of the scapular spine in 89% of cadaveric dissections.[1] The fourth muscle is the teres minor; its origin is the lateral border of the scapula, and its insertion is the lower aspect of the greater tuberosity. It is innervated by the axillary nerve (C5,6).

The rotator interval between the subscapularis and the supraspinatus tendons is reinforced by the coracohumeral ligament. In this region, fibrous slips from the tendons of the subscapularis and supraspinatus combine to form a sheath around the long head of the biceps tendon. The cuff tendons inserting into the greater tuberosity fuse into a tendinous aponeurosis.[2] The pattern of intersecting fibers is such that the forces generated by an individual cuff muscle are transmitted to the tendons of adjacent cuff muscles. These forces are not isolated only to that muscle's attachment to the humerus but to the attachments of adjacent tendons as well. This interconnected arrangement of the rotator cuff tendon insertions undoubtedly influences the ultimate configuration and complexity of cuff tears.

On the microscopic level, the insertion complex of the subscapularis and supraspinatus tendons has been described as a five-layer structure[2] (Fig. 1). Layer one is composed of the superficial fibers of the coracohumeral ligament. Layer two is the primary portion of the cuff tendons and is seen as closely packed parallel tendon fibers grouped in large bundles extending directly from the muscle bellies to the insertion on the humerus. Layer three is a similarly thick tendinous structure with tendon fascicles that are smaller and less uniformly oriented than layer two. Layer four contains the deep extension of the coracohumeral ligament, which has thick bands of collagen fibers running perpendicular to the primary fiber orientation of the cuff tendons. This layer likely assists in the distribution of forces between different tendons and may explain why normal kinematics may be maintained even in the presence of large tendon defects. Layer five is the true capsular layer, which forms a continuous cylinder from the glenoid to the humerus in which fibers are randomly oriented.

This multilayer structure has also been described by Gohlke and associates[3] (Fig. 2). They speculated that because of the various fiber orientations and distinct layers within the capsular complex, significant shear stresses exist that may play a role in cuff tears. Furthermore, the intratendinous interdigitations and variations in the cuff structure probably are important to the pattern of propagation of partial thickness and intrasubstance tears.

The vascular anatomy of the rotator cuff has always been the subject of focused interest because of its suggested role in the pathogenesis of rotator cuff tears. Blood reaches the rotator cuff from several arterial sources. The posterior circumflex humeral artery and suprascapular arteries form an interlacing arcade over the posterior cuff and constitute the major blood supply to the teres minor and the infraspinatus.[4] The anterior circumflex humeral artery travels at the inferior border of the subscapularis muscle, supplying portions of

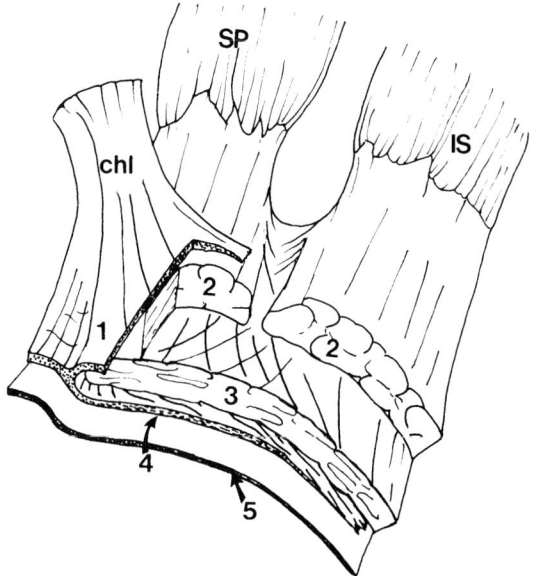

FIGURE 1

Schematic diagram of a dissection sectioned transversely at various sites in the supraspinatus (SP) and infraspinatus (IS) tendons and capsule of the shoulder. The orientations of the fascicles in the numbered layers are indicated by the lines on their upper surfaces. Layer 1 is composed of superficial fibers that overlie the cuff tendons and extend from the coracoid process to the greater tuberosity. These fibers form an extension of the coracohumeral ligament (chl). Layers 2 and 3 contain the fibers of the supraspinatus and infraspinatus tendons. In Layer 4 the fibers make up the deep extension of the coracohumeral ligament. Layer 5 is the true joint capsule of the shoulder, which forms a continuous fibrous cylinder extending from the glenoid labrum to the neck of the humerus. The synovial lining of the capsule is in direct contact with the articular surface of the humeral head. The orientation of the fibers within the capsule is quite variable and is not identified in this diagram. (Reproduced with permission from Clark JM, Harryman DT II: Tendons, ligaments, and capsule of the rotator cuff: Gross and microscopic anatomy. *J Bone Joint Surg* 1992;74A:713–725.)

the anterosuperior cuff in conjunction with the thoracoacromial artery[4] and a variable distal branch that Rothman and Parke[5] called the suprahumeral artery. The acromial branch of the thoracoacromial artery usually supplies the supraspinatus muscle.

CORACOACROMIAL ARCH ANATOMY

The coracoacromial arch comprises the bony acromion, the coracoacromial ligament, and the

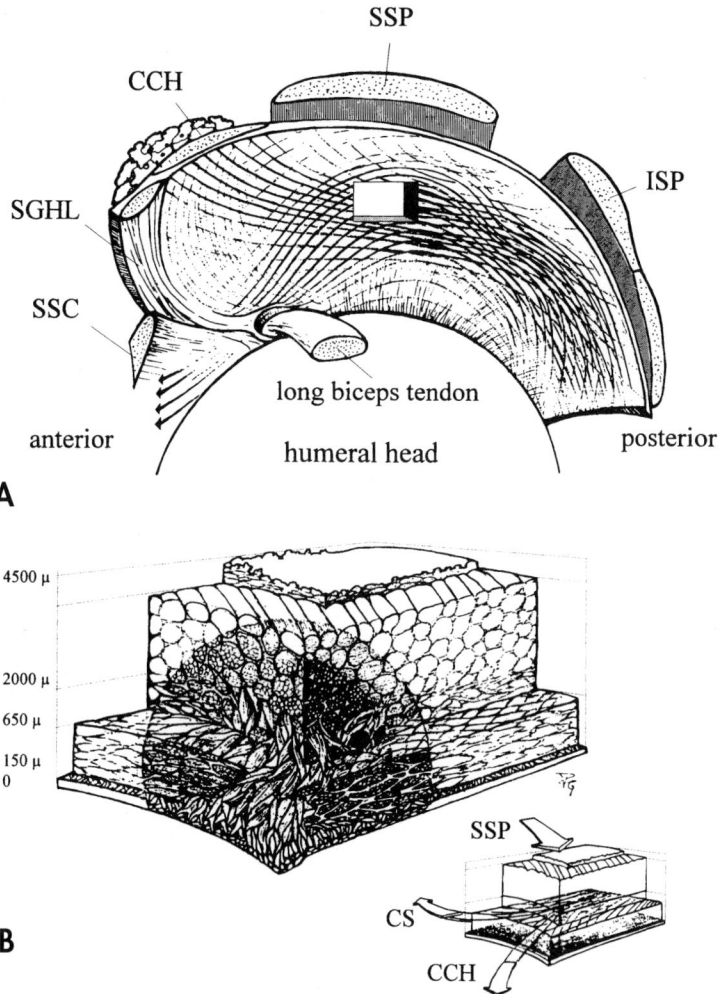

FIGURE 2
Structure of the superior complex. **A,** View of superior capsule from articular side. SSP = supraspinatus, ISP = infraspinatus, SGHL = superior glenohumeral ligament, CCH = coracohumeral ligament. A small block of tissue has been removed. **B,** Diagram of tissue from block in top showing three-dimensional reconstruction of intermingling of collagen fiber bundles of capsule. cs = circular system of fiber bundles. (Reproduced with permission from Gohlke F, Essigkrug B, Schmitz F: The pattern of the collagen fiber bundles of the capsule of the glenohumeral joint. *J Shoulder Elbow Surg* 1994;3:111–128.)

coracoid process. This structure forms the roof of the space, known as the supraspinatus outlet, through which the supraspinatus tendon passes. Because of its position directly above the rotator cuff, the coracoacromial arch has been implicated in rotator cuff pathology.

Typically, the acromion has two or three centers of ossification that fuse by age 22 years. Failure of the ossification of the acromion leads to a persistent unfused acromial epiphysis (os acromiale). In a radiologic survey of 1,800 shoulders, Liberson[6] observed an overall incidence of os acromiale of 1.4% with 62% being bilateral.[7] Folliasson[8] classified the lesion into four distinct types anatomically as pre-, meso-, meta-, and basiacromion, based on their embryologic origin.

3

The coracoacromial ligament is triangular, and runs from the lateral aspect of the coracoid to the anteroinferior acromion.[9–11] Holt and Allibone[12] classified the ligament into three types: (1) quadrangular; (2) Y-shaped, consisting of both lateral and medial bands; and (3) one broad band. Anteroinferior acromial spurs tend to develop by ossification of the coracoacromial ligament.[13]

ETIOLOGY OF TENDON FAILURE

A consensus has emerged that rotator cuff disease is multifactorial, including extrinsic factors, such as subacromial and internal impingement, tensile overload, and repetitive stress, and intrinsic factors, such as poor vascularity, alterations in material properties and matrix composition, and aging.[14–19]

TENDON DEGENERATION

In the healthy, young cuff, the tendon is stronger than the bone, and avulsion fractures of the greater tuberosity are more common than tendon tears. Thus, even when trauma is involved, it generally is believed that most full cuff tears occur through tendons already weakened by degeneration.[20,21] It is the nature of this degeneration which is debated.[22] Questions to be considered are why is the supraspinatus tendon usually the initial site of tear formation,[23,24] and why is the articular side more commonly involved in partial tears?

Microinjection studies of the vascular anatomy of the rotator cuff classically have supported the notion of a "hypovascular zone" within the tendinous portion of the supraspinatus.[5,25–27] Microvascular studies have shown that vascularity is diminished in cuff tissues from older individuals as compared to tissue from younger individuals, which is consistent with the observed pattern of age-related tendon degeneration.[28] Vascularity may also be transiently decreased due to dynamic factors. Rathbun and Macnab[27] noted that the blood supply of the supraspinatus tendon depended on arm position, becoming hypovascular when the microinjection was given with the arm in adduction. Furthermore, pressure studies of the subacromial space demonstrate that lifting

a 1-kg weight can increase subacromial contact pressures enough to block microcirculation, suggesting a dynamic vascular compromise that is related to functional activities of daily living.[29] Other microinjection studies have revealed an adequate blood supply, particularly to the bursal side, with relative hypovascularity on the articular side.[30–32]

However, other studies have disputed the role of hypovascularity in causing tendon defects. Brooks and associates[33] could not find an area of hypovascularity in the supraspinatus tendon. Swiontkowski and associates,[34,35] using microvascular techniques with laser Doppler flowmetry in living patients, have noted hypervascularity in the supraspinatus tendon. Thus, the role of hypovascularity as a pathogenic factor in degenerative rotator cuff tears remains unclear.

The possibility that intrinsic tendon degeneration might be related to variations in tendon composition and material properties has been investigated. Itoi and associates[36] noted variations in material properties within the supraspinatus tendon (Fig. 3). Nakajima and associates[37] compared the material properties of the articular surface of the supraspinatus tendon versus the bursal surface. The bursal side showed a significantly lower modulus of elasticity and higher ultimate strain, from which the authors concluded that the joint side of the tendon was more susceptible to mechanical failure than the bursal side at similar loads.

Soslowsky and associates[38] injected rat supraspinatus tendons with collagenase to simulate intrinsic degeneration. However, loss of material properties only persisted when a mechanical insult was added. Nirschl[39] has proposed that the degenerative tendinopathy seen in the cuff is similar to that which occurs in lateral epicondylitis or Achilles tendon ruptures, and represents angiofibroblastic dysplasia. Although often described as chronic tendinitis, true inflammation is rarely seen.[39]

It has been suggested that tendon degeneration might result from an incomplete or inappropriate repair response. Repetitive microtrauma[40] and tensile loads might cause "microtears," which

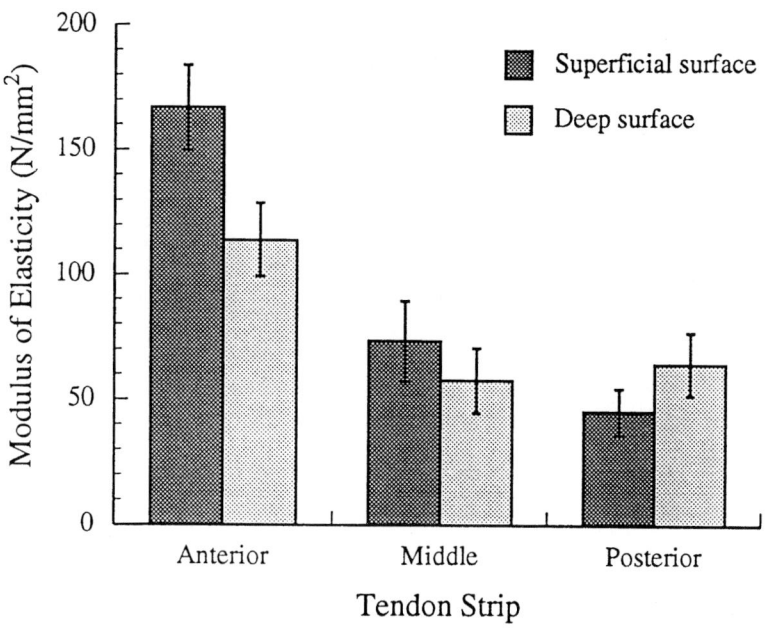

FIGURE 3

Modulus of elasticity of the supraspinatus tendon by region. The anterior strip showed a significantly greater modulus of elasticity than the middle and posterior strips (p < 0.0001). There were no significant differences between the superficial and deep surfaces. The bars indicate the mean ± SEM. (Reproduced with permission from Itoi E, Berglund LJ, Grabowski JJ, et al: Tensile properties of the supraspinatus tendon. *J Orthop Res* 1995;13:578–584.

could overwhelm the healing response, causing fiber disorganization and stress concentrations. Matrix changes may also result. In patients with cuff disease, gene expression for the core protein of aggrecan has been found to be increased in the supraspinatus as compared to the subscapularis, suggesting that subacromial impingement may have induced the tenocytes to shift the matrix to one better suited to resisting compression,[41] thereby rendering the tendon more vulnerable to tensile failure.

IMPINGEMENT

Sixty years ago, Meyer[42,43] implicated mechanical attrition under the acromion in the pathogenesis of both rotator cuff degeneration and biceps tendon rupture. In 1972, Neer[44,45] proposed that differences in the size and shape of the structures of the coracoacromial arch were relevant to the development of rotator cuff pathology. He identified the anterior third of the undersurface of the

acromion, the coracoacromial ligament, and the acromioclavicular joint as areas that may compress and damage the cuff tendons.

Bigliani and associates[46] demonstrated an association between qualitative changes in the shape of the acromion and the incidence of full-thickness rotator cuff tears. In a study of 140 cadavers, three distinct types of acromial morphology were identified by lateral radiographs tilted 10° cephalad (supraspinatus outlet view).[47] Those types included a type I, or flat acromion in 17%; type II, or curved acromion in 43%; and type III, or hooked acromion, in 40% (Fig. 4). There was a significant increase in full-thickness rotator cuff tearing with the type III acromial shape, in acromions with anterior spurs, and in acromions with a greater angle of anterior slope. In a subsequent clinical study, Morrison and Bigliani[48] found that in those patients with a positive arthrogram, 80% had a type III acromion.

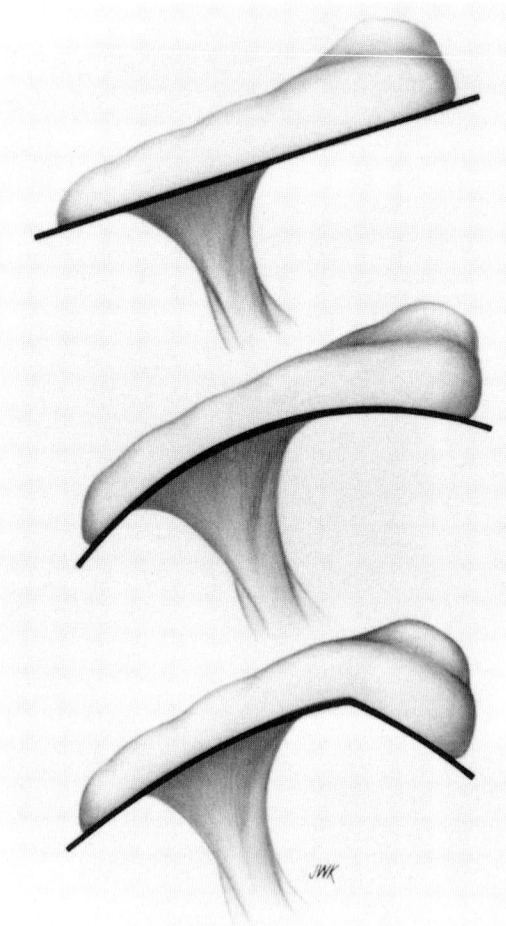

FIGURE 4
Bigliani classification of acromial morphology. (Reproduced with permission from Frymoyer JW (ed): *Orthopaedic Knowledge Update 4*. Rosemont, IL, American Academy of Orthopaedic Surgeons, 1993, p 308.)

Wuh and Snyder[49] modified the Bigliani classification by addressing acromial thickness as well as acromial shape. The acromial thickness was measured at the junction of the anterior to middle third of the acromion. Type A acromions are less than 8 mm thick, type B between 8 and 12 mm, and type C acromions are greater than 12 mm (Fig. 5). Acromial shape and length have also been studied by Edelson and Taitz[50] who found that the more horizontal the acromion, the greater the degenerative changes. In addition, they noted

increased degenerative changes with increased length of the acromion. Although several reports have noted the association of unfused acromial epiphyses with rotator cuff tears,[50–52] there is little evidence to suggest that this condition actually predisposes the shoulder to the development of a rotator cuff tear.

It has been disputed whether acromial morphology is a cause of tendon degeneration, or whether cuff failure occurs first, allowing the head to ascend, abrade the acromion, and cause changes in acromial shape secondarily. Nicholson and associates[53] found no significant change in acromial morphology with age in a study of 420 scapulae in 10-year age cohorts from 21 to 70 years of age from the Cleveland Museum of Natural History, suggesting that acromial architecture is a primary anatomic characteristic. Thus, certain shapes may be risk factors for the development of rotator cuff disease. This study was careful to separately evaluate anteroinferior spurs in the coracoacromial ligament from acromial shape. Indeed, spur formation increased dramatically with age.

These spurs, essentially osteophytes that form on the anterior third of the acromion at the insertion of the coracoacromial ligament, can further decrease the volume available for supraspinatus tendon excursion.[54–56] Aoki and associates[57] measured the slope of the acromion on lateral radiographs of 130 cadaver shoulders. They found that acromions with spur formation had a flatter slope (Fig. 5) with increased pitting on the surface of the greater tuberosity. This flattening of the slope of the acromion may produce impingement of the rotator cuff between the acromion and the superior surface of the humeral greater tuberosity, leading to degenerative changes. When comparing asymptomatic patients with patients having stage II impingement, the latter group had a statistically flatter slope.

Zuckerman and associates[58] used four reference points and three-dimensional computer modeling to quantify the area under the coracoacromial arch as well as the supraspinatus outlet. The results were correlated with the presence, location, and size of rotator cuff tears. The group with rotator

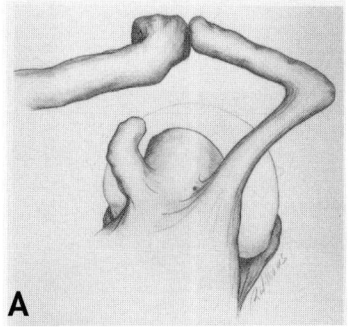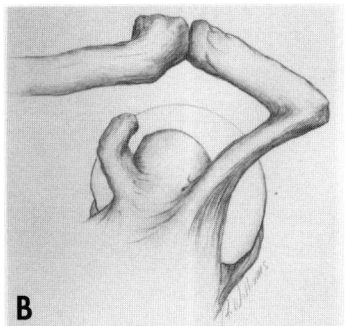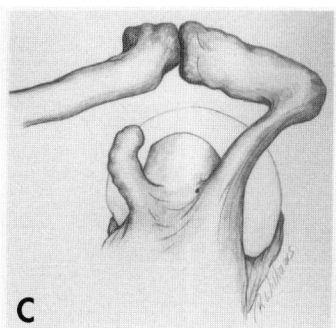

FIGURE 5
A, Type A arch: Acromion less than 8-mm thick. **B,** Type B arch: Acromion between 8 and 12 mm thick. **C,** Type C arch: Acromion greater than 12 mm thick. (Reproduced with permission from Snyder SJ, Wuh HC: Arthroscopic management of the rotator cuff and superior labrum anterior posterior lesion. *Oper Tech Orthop* 1991;1:207–220.)

cuff tears had a smaller gap between the humeral head and the coracoacromial ligament, a smaller supraspinatus outlet, and flatter acromial tilt.

The manner in which the coracoacromial arch might contact the rotator cuff tendons has been investigated. Burns and Whipple[59] made qualitative visual observations of subacromial contact in articulated cadaveric shoulders. They found that contact by the anterior tip of the acromion on the supraspinatus tendon and the greater tuberosity was greatest in the middle ranges of humeral elevation, 60° to 120°. Similar findings were noted with dye compression and pressure-sensitive film.[60,61]

A recent finite element model of the stress environment in the supraspinatus tendon showed that extrinsic compression by subacromial impingement generates high stress concentrations, sufficient to cause a tear, in and around the critical zone of the supraspinatus tendon.[62] High stress due to impingement could be generated on the bursal side, on the articular side, or within the tendon, as might be expected when a soft tissue (tendon) is compressed between two bones (humerus and acromion). This fact illustrates the error of the traditionally simplistic reasoning that only bursal-sided partial tears could be initiated by subacromial impingement.

More recently, Flatow and associates[63] used optical stereophotogrammetric techniques to assess subacromial contact. The principal advantage of this technique is that it allows measurements to be made without disrupting the joint capsule or subacromial space, thus more accurately representing the native anatomic state. The acromion comes closest to the cuff tendons between 60° and 120° of elevation, with contact focused at the supraspinatus insertion (Fig. 6). When internally rotated 20°, more shoulders were in contact than in the neutral position. Also noted was increased contact with shoulders having type III acromions than with other types.

The data collected also permitted computer simulation of acromioplasty.[64] The three-dimensional shape of the acromion was altered by three algorithms: (1) removing any anteroinferior ridges (spurs); (2) flattening the anterior third of the acromion; and (3) flattening the entire acromion flush with the posterior acromion as described by Caspari and Thal.[65] Impingement, defined as focused acromial contact compressing the supraspinatus insertion, was eliminated in 50% of the specimens by just removing anterior ridges. Flattening of the anterior third of the acromion successfully removed impingement in 100% of the specimens. Total flattening was thus deemed unnecessary to eliminate impingement, and, in fact, often destroyed the broad pattern of subacromial contact over the other cuff tendons and humeral head. This diffuse contact, termed *buffering* in the study, was thought to have a passive, stabilizing role against superior humeral ascent.

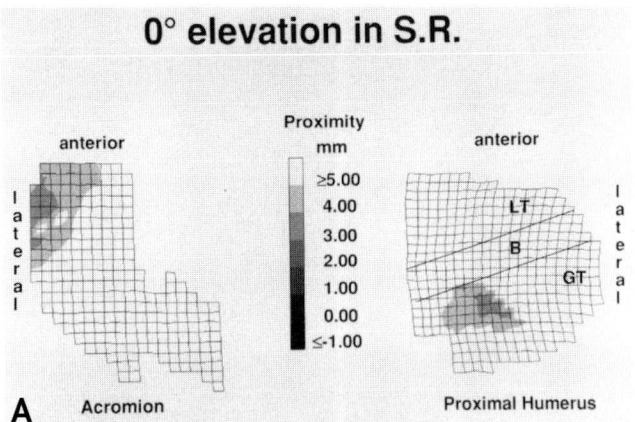

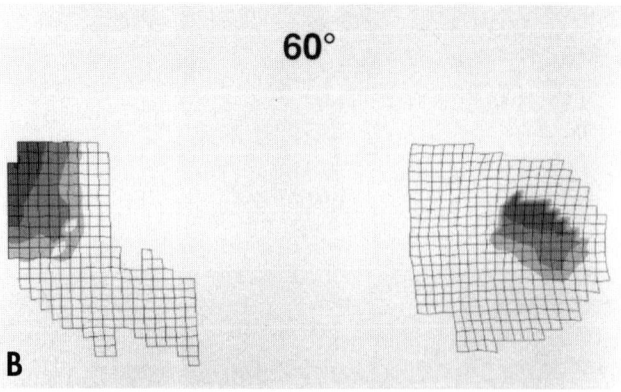

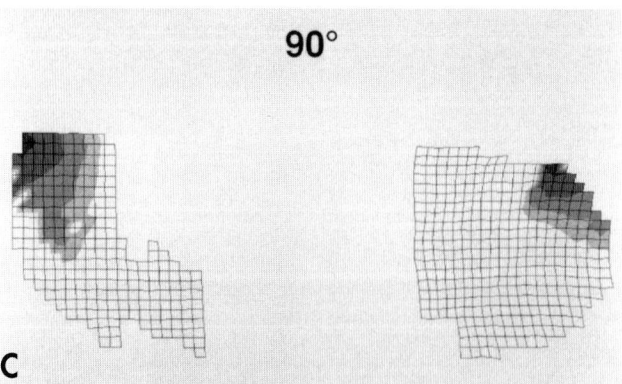

FIGURE 6

A, Subacromial contact patterns for a right shoulder at 0° of arm elevation in the starting rotation (SR). Gray levels represent proximity of one surface to the other in millimeters. B = biceps tendon region, GT = greater tuberosity, LT = lesser tuberosity. **B,** Same shoulder at 60° of elevation. **C,** Same shoulder at 90° of elevation. (Reproduced with permission from Flatow EL, Soslowsky LJ, Ticker JB, et al: Excursion of the rotator cuff under the acromion: Patterns of subacromial contact. *Am J Sports Med* 1994;22:779–788.)

Unfortunately, contact by the coracoacromial arch on the underlying humerus and rotator cuff has been only thought of as potentially deleterious. However, increased attention has been given recently to the role of the arch as an important passive stabilizer against superior humeral subluxation; it may be the last restraint left when the rotator cuff is no longer functioning to dynamically center the humeral head in the glenoid. This has been confirmed by cadaver studies.[66–68] Indeed, Wiley[69] reported superior humeral dislocation in patients who had undergone coracoacromial arch decompression without repair of massive rotator cuff tears (Fig. 7). Because of such concerns, at the time of repair of massive rotator cuff tears Flatow and associates have used reattachment of the coracoacromial ligament after a conservative acromioplasty to preserve a buffering role for the coracoacromial arch[70] (Fig. 8), and have even reconstructed an arch in some cases of failed repairs.[71]

Thus it seems likely that subacromial contact, when abnormal and focused on the supraspina-tus insertion, may cause tendon wear and injury, but that it also is part of a normal stabilizing mechanism.

ROTATOR CUFF KINEMATICS

The primary function of the rotator cuff is to act as a humeral head depressor and dynamic stabilizer of the glenohumeral joint, creating a fulcrum from which the deltoid can elevate the arm.[72] The rotator cuff muscles additionally provide rotation of the humeral head. Classically, the infraspinatus and teres minor have been described as primary external rotators of the arm, providing as much as 80% of the external rotation force.[30] The subscapularis acts as an internal rotator as well as a powerful dynamic barrier to anterior displacement of the humeral head,[73] whereas the supraspinatus provides approximately 50% of the torque output in shoulder elevation.[74]

More recent studies have shown a much more intricate interplay of the rotator cuff muscles in both simple and complex movements of the glenohumeral joint. The contributions and

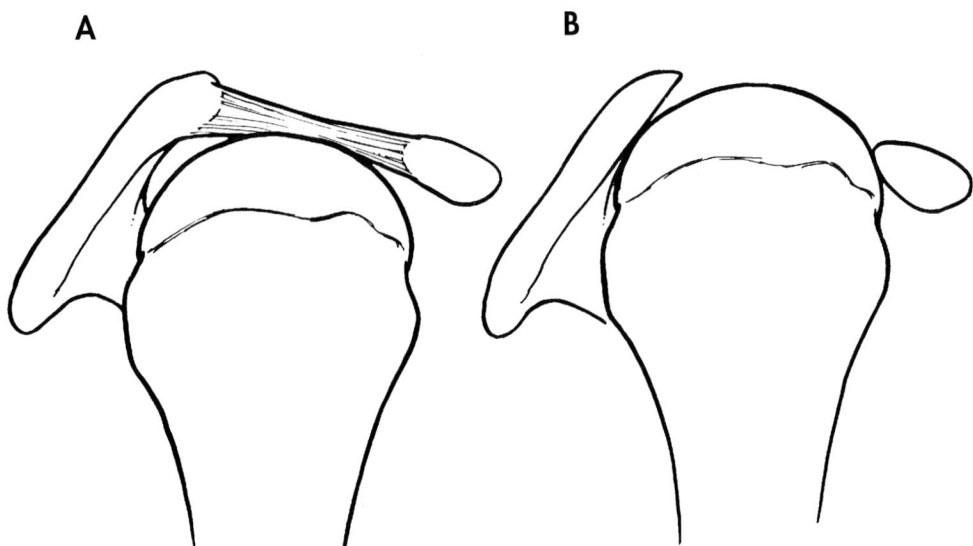

A **B**

FIGURE 7
A, With a massive rotator cuff tear, the humeral head rises superiorly, resting under the coracoacromial arch. **B,** Resection of the anterior acromion and coracoacromial ligament can lead to anterosuperior humeral head subluxation if the rotator cuff is unrepaired, retorn, or nonfunctional. (Reproduced with permission from Bigliani LU, Codd TP, Flatow EL: Arthroscopic coracoacromial ligament resection. *Tech Orthop* 1994;9:95–97.)

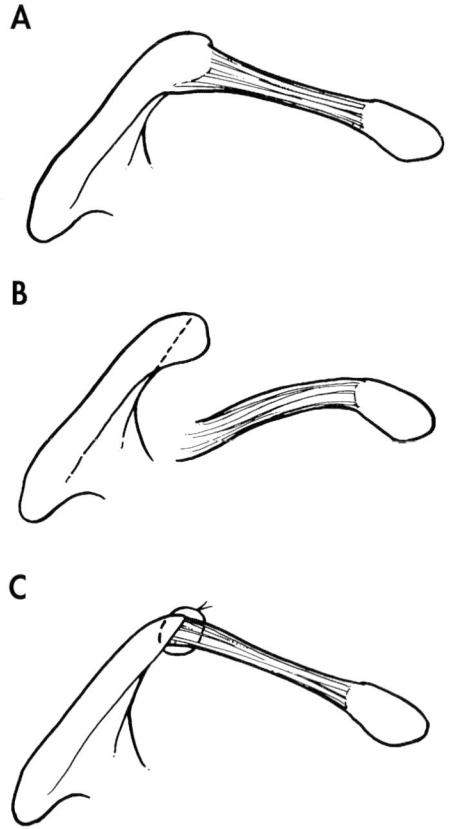

FIGURE 8
Modified acromioplasty to preserve the coracoacromial (CA) ligament. **A,** The coracoacromial ligament insertion is incised, preserving as much length as possible. **B,** A conservative anterior acromioplasty is performed to make smooth the undersurface of the acromion. **C,** After completion of the tendon repair, the CA ligament is repaired to the anteromedial aspect of the acromion with transosseous sutures. Preservation of the CA ligament is reserved for cases in which it is felt that tendon repair will not restore active humeral head depression. (Reproduced with permission from Bigliani LU, Codd TP, Flatow EL: Arthroscopic coracoacromial ligament resection. *Tech Orthop* 1994;9:95–97.)

capacities of the individual muscles, even parts of muscles, depend on moment arms, line of action, and glenohumeral joint position. Understanding those contributions clarifies the roles of the rotator cuff muscles in cuff pathology, repair, and rehabilitation.

Various biomechanical, kinematic, and mathematical models have been developed to assess the role of the rotator cuff in both normal and abnormal conditions. The role of cuff muscles in abduction and rotation has been deduced from muscle geometry and orientation,[75] and from electromyographic studies.[76–79] Otis and associates[80] studied changes in moment arms of the rotator cuff and deltoid muscles with abduction and rotation using a cadaveric model. They found that the abductor moment arm of the anterior portion of the supraspinatus decreased with internal rotation, whereas that of the posterior portion of the supraspinatus decreased with external rotation. The infraspinatus was both an external rotator and abductor. Internal rotation markedly enhanced the effectiveness of the superior portion of the infraspinatus as an abductor (Fig. 9), whereas abduction reduced the effectiveness of the superior portion of the infraspinatus as an external rotator. The subscapularis was an internal rotator with an abductor moment arm greatest for the superior portion of the subscapularis. External rotation increased the ability of the superior portion of the subscapularis to elevate the arm.

The effect of cuff failure has been investigated with biomechanical models in an attempt to understand the clinical variability. Many shoulders with massive tears appear to have normal kinematics, whereas others may be severely impaired. Burkhart[81] proposed a model in which a balance of forces anteriorly and posteriorly might preserve stability, whereas a thick free edge of the cuff tear might transmit stresses around the tear in a manner analogous to the cable in a suspension bridge. Cadaver models have been used to simulate cuff tears, and it generally has been found that supraspinatus tears may increase the deltoid force needed to lift the arm but don't alter the kinematics.[82,83]

Flatow and associates[84] recently developed a cadaveric model that quantitatively examined both the active (rotator cuff and biceps) and passive (coracoacromial arch) stabilizers and related the effects of those factors to rotator cuff decompression and surgical repair. When a full-thickness defect in the supraspinatus tendon was created,

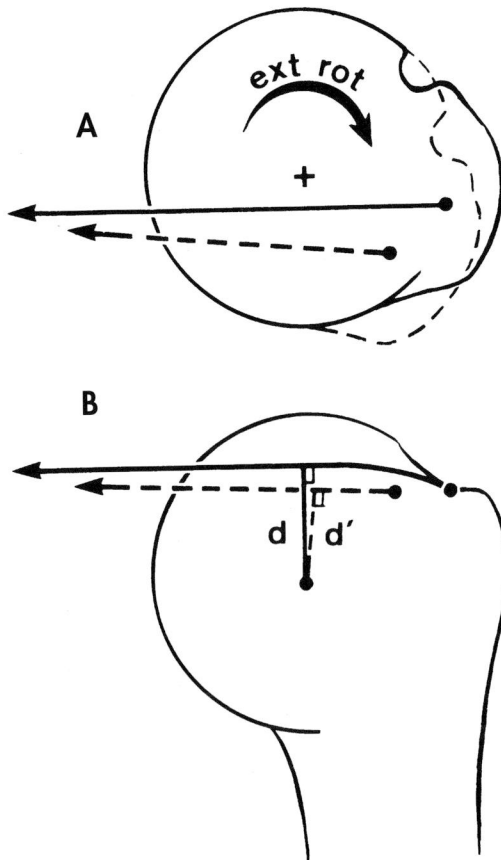

FIGURE 9

Change in moment-arm of the infraspinatus with rotation. As the insertion of the infraspinatus moves posteriorly with external rotation (**A**), the tendon drops from its more superior location on the humeral head (**B**), so that its line of action is closer to the axis of abduction. The effect is a reduction of the moment-arm length from d to d´. The initial position of the infraspinatus is shown as a solid line and the final position as a dashed line. (Reproduced with permission from Otis C, Jiang C, Wickiewicz TL, Peterson MG, Warren RF, Satner TJ: Changes in the moment arms of the rotator cuff and deltoid muscles with abduction and rotation. *J Bone Joint Surg* 1994;76A:667–676.)

centering of the head was impaired, and some of the arms could not be elevated. In contrast, when pain inhibition was simulated by leaving the supraspinatus intact but applying no force to it, the center of the humeral head translated superiorly, but to a lesser degree, and full active elevation was possible in each shoulder. This difference

was proposed to be due to the passive "spacer effect" of the tendon, which restrains superior humeral translation and provides a smooth surface continuous with the greater tuberosity, which can glide below the acromion in the critical midrange of motion.

There was a progressive and statistically significant increase in superior translation with increasing size of simulated cuff defects. Tendon repair restored kinematics in all cases. This model likely only represents the *potential* of cuff repair, because in the clinical situation there is usually some degree of irreversible muscle atrophy, so that full force may not be restored to the repaired tendon as it is in the cadaver model simulation. The superior translation seen with large cuff defects could be reduced by the application of a force to the intact biceps tendon. Often, this stabilizing effect restored full active elevation despite large cuff defects. These findings suggest that force in the tendon of the long head of the biceps, whether active[85–87] or just due to passive muscle-tendon stretch,[88–90] and the spacer effect of the tendon, help to stabilize the humeral head with a massive cuff tear. This supports many clinicians' impressions that the sacrifice of the biceps at surgical reconstruction of a rotator cuff tear may impair the fulcrum for arm elevation.[88,91,92]

The study also addressed the function of the coracoacromial ligament in stabilizing the shoulder. Transsection of the coracoacromial ligament in this model, afer the creation of massive cuff tears, allowed for the largest superior humeral subluxations. This subluxation seemed to occur by two mechanisms: loss of the "buffering" contact by the undersurface of the coracoacromial ligament on the ascending head, and loss of the "tethering" between the coracoid and the anterior acromial tip allowing the acromion to deform upward. This springing open of the coracoacromial gap allowed marked anterosuperior migration.

As noted previously, the authors drew a distinction between impingement, defined as a focused contact by the anteroinferior acromion and the coracoacromial ligament insertion on the supraspinatus insertion, and buffering, defined as the broad area of contact under the entire acromial undersurface. The coracoacromial ligament was thus viewed as an important passive stabilizer[23,39,70,84] and often the final passive restraint to anterosuperior humeral migration when the dynamic head centering function of the rotator cuff was compromised by tears.

CONCLUSION

A consensus is finally emerging that rotator cuff disease is a multifactorial disorder. Extrinsic factors, such as the morphology of the coracoacromial arch, kinematic abnormalities, tensile overload, and repetitive use injuries, and intrinsic factors, such as altered tendon vascular supply, regional variation in material properties, and ultrastructural collagen fiber alterations, exist. Once tears occur, kinematics may be altered in complex ways. A major theme of recent research has been the stabilizing role of the coracoacromial arch. The previous discussion has presented much of the current information on the anatomic, biomechanical, and kinematic features of the coracoacromial arch and the underlying rotator cuff.

REFERENCES

1. Bigliani LU, Dalsey RM, McCann PD, April EW: An anatomical study of the suprascapular nerve. *Arthroscopy* 1990;6:301–305.

2. Clark JM, Harryman DT II: Tendons, ligaments, and capsule of the rotator cuff: Gross and microscopic anatomy. *J Bone Joint Surg* 1992; 74A:713–725.

3. Gohlke F, Daum P, Eulert J: Abstract: The stabilizing function of the capsule of the glenohumeral joint and the corresponding role of the coracoacromial arch. *J Shoulder Elbow Surg* 1994;3:S24.

4. Gerber C, Schneeberger AG, Vinh TS: The arterial vascularization of the humeral head: An anatomical study. *J Bone Joint Surg* 1990; 72A:1486–1494.

5. Rothman RH, Parke WW: The vascular anatomy of the rotator cuff. *Clin Orthop* 1965;41:176–186.

6. Liberson F: Os acromiale: A contested anomaly. *J Bone Joint Surg* 1937;19:683–689.

7. Edelson JG, Zuckerman J, Hershkovitz I: Os acromiale: Anatomy and surgical implications. *J Bone Joint Surg* 1993;75B:551–555.

8. Folliasson A: Un cas d'os acromial. *Rev d'Orthop* 1933;20:533–538.

9. Sakar K, Taine W, Uhthoff HK: The ultrastructure of the coracoacromial ligament in patients with chronic impingement syndrome. *Clin Orthop* 1990;254:49–54.

10. Soslowsky LJ, An CH, DeBano CM, et al: The coracoacromial ligament: In situ load and viscoelastic properties in rotator cuff disease. *Clin Orthop* 1996;330:40–44.

11. Soslowsky LJ, An CH, Johnston SP, et al: Geometric and mechanical properties of the coracoacromial ligament and their relationship to rotator cuff disease. *Clin Orthop* 1994; 304:10–17.

12. Holt EM, Allibone RO: Anatomic variants of the coracoacromial ligament. *J Shoulder Elbow Surg* 1995;4:370–375.

13. Flatow EL, Fealy S, April EW, O'Flynn HM, Armengol-Barallat J, Bigliani LU: Abstract: The coracoacromial ligament: Anatomy, morphology and a study of acromial enthesopathy. *J Shoulder Elbow Surg* 1996;5:S60.

14. Blevins FT, Djurasovic M, Flatow EL, Vogel KG: Biology of the rotator cuff tendon. *Orthop Clin North Am* 1997;28:1–16.

15. Cofield RH: Rotator cuff disease of the shoulder. *J Bone Joint Surg* 1985;67A:974–979.

16. Fu FH, Harner CD,* Klein AH: Shoulder impingement syndrome: A critical review. *Clin Orthop* 1991;269:162–173.

17. Soslowsky LJ, Carpenter JE, Bucchieri JS, Flatow EL: Biomechanics of the rotator cuff. *Orthop Clin North Am* 1997;28:17–30.

18. Uhthoff HK, Drummond DI, Sakar K, et al: The role of impingement syndrome: A clinical, radiological, and histological study. *Int Orthop* 1988;12:97.

19. Uhthoff HJ, Sana S: Pathology of failure of the rotator cuff tendon. *Orthop Clin North Am* 1997;28:31–41.

20. Wilson CL: Experimental degeneration of the supraspinatus tendon. *J Bone Joint Surg* 1948; 30A:769–773.

21. Wilson CL, Duff GL: Pathologic study of degeneration and rupture of the supraspinatus tendon. *Arch Surg* 1943;47:121–135.

22. Ogata S, Uhthoff: Acromial enthesopathy and rotator cuff tears. *Clin Orthop* 1990;254:39–48.

23. Codman EA (ed): *The Shoulder: Rupture of the Supraspinatus Tendon and Other Lesions In or About the Subacromial Bursa.* Boston, MA, Thomas Todd, 1934.

24. McLaughlin HL: Ruptures of the rotator cuff. *J Bone Joint Surg* 1962;23A:979–983.

25. Lindblom K, Palmer I: Ruptures of the tendon aponeurosis of the shoulder joint: The so-called supraspinatus ruptures. *Acta Chir Scand* 1939; 82:133–142.

26. Moseley HF, Goldie I: The arterial pattern of the rotator cuff of the shoulder. *J Bone Joint Surg* 1963;45B:780–789.

27. Rathbun JB, Macnab I: The microvascular pattern of the rotator cuff. *J Bone Joint Surg* 1970; 52B:540–553.

28. Fukuda H, Hamada K, Yamanaka K: Pathology and pathogenesis of bursal-side rotator cuff tears viewed from en bloc histologic sections. *Clin Orthop* 1990;254:75–80.

29. Sigholm G, Styf J, Korner L, Herberts P: Pressure recordings in the subacromial bursa. *J Orthop Res* 1988;6:123–128.

30. Iannotti JP (ed): *Rotator Cuff Disorders: Evaluation and Treatment.* Park Ridge, IL, American Academy of Orthopaedic Surgeons, 1991.

31. Uhthoff HK, Kumagai J, Sarkar K, Lohr J, Murnaghan P: Abstract: Morphologic evidence of healing in torn human rotator cuffs. *J Bone Joint Surg* 1992;74B(suppl 3):293–294.

32. Uhthoff HK, Lohr J, Sarkar K: The pathogenesis of rotator cuff tears, in Takagishi N (ed): *The Shoulder: Proceedings of the Third International Conference on Surgery of the Shoulder.* Tokyo, Japan, Professional Graduate Services, 1987, pp 211–212.

33. Brooks CH, Revell WJ, Heatley FW: A quantitative histological study of the vascularity of the rotator cuff tendon. *J Bone Joint Surg* 1992; 74B:151–153.

34. Swiontkowski MF, Iannotti JP, Boulas HJ, Esterhai JL: Intraoperative assessment of rotator cuff vascularity using laser Doppler flowmetry, in Post M, Morrey BF, Hawkins RJ (eds): *Surgery of the Shoulder.* St. Louis, MO, Mosby-Year Book, 1990, pp 208–212.

35. Swiontkowski M, Iannotti JP, Esterhai JL, Boulas HJ: Intraoperative assessment of rotator cuff vascularity using laser Doppler flowmetry. Proceedings of the 56th Annual Meeting of the American Academy of Orthopaedic Surgeons, Las Vegas, NV. Park Ridge, IL, American Academy of Orthopaedic Surgeons, 1989, p 73.

36. Itoi E, Berglund LJ, Grabowski JJ, et al: Tensile properties of the supraspinatus tendon. *J Orthop Res* 1995;13:578–584.

37. Nakajima T, Rokuuma N, Hamada K, et al: Histologic and biomechanical characteristics of the supraspinatus tendon: Reference to rotator cuff tearing. *J Shoulder Elbow Surg* 1994;3:79–87.

38. Soslowsky LJ, Carpenter JE, DeBano CM, Banerji I, Moalli MR: Development and use of an animal model for investigations on rotator cuff disease. *J Shoulder Elbow Surg* 1996;5:383–392.

39. Nirschl RP: Rotator cuff surgery, in Barr JS Jr (ed): *Instructional Course Lectures XXXVIII.* Park Ridge, IL, American Academy of Orthopaedic Surgeons, 1989, pp 447–462.

40. Cotton RE, Rideout DF: Tears of the humeral rotator cuff: A radiological and pathological necropsy survey. *J Bone Joint Surg* 1964; 46B;314–328.

41. Flatow EL, Djurasovic M, Bigliani LU, Ratcliffe A: Abstract: Variation of proteoglycan gene expression in rotator cuff tendons. *J Shoulder Elbow Surg* 1997;6:220.

42. Meyer AW: The minute anatomy of attrition lesions. *J Bone Joint Surg* 1931;13:341–348.

43. Meyer AW: Chronic functional lesions of the shoulder. *Arch Surg* 1937;35:646–674.

44. Neer CS II: Anterior acromioplasty for chronic impingement in the shoulder: A preliminary report. *J Bone Joint Surg* 1972;54A:41–50.

45. Neer CS II (ed): Cuff tears, biceps lesions, and impingement, in *Shoulder Reconstruction.* Philadelphia, PA, WB Saunders, 1990, pp 41–142.

46. Bigliani LU, Morrison DS, April EW: The morphology of the acromion and its relationship to rotator cuff tears. *Orthop Trans* 1986;10:228.

47. Neer CS II, Poppen NK: Supraspinatus outlet. *Orthop Trans* 1987;11:234.

48. Morrison DS, Bigliani LU: The clinical significance of variations in acromial morphology. *Orthop Trans* 1987;11:234.

49. Wuh HCK, Snyder SJ: A modified classification of the supraspinatus outlet view based on the configuration and the anatomic thickness of the acromion. *Orthop Trans* 1992;16:767.

50. Edelson JG, Taitz C: Anatomy of the coraco-acromial arch: Relationship to degeneration of the acromion. *J Bone Joint Surg* 1992; 74B:589–594.

51. Bigliani LU, Norris TR, Fischer J, Neer CS: The relationship between the unfused acromial epiphysis and subacromial lesions. *Orthop Trans* 1983;7:138.

52. Mudge MK, Fryman CK, Wood VE: Rotator cuff tears associated with os acromiale. *J Bone Joint Surg* 1984;66A:427–429.

53. Nicholson GP, Goodman DA, Flatow EL, Bigliani LU: The acromion: Morphologic condition and age-related changes. A study of 420 scapulas. *J Shoulder Elbow Surg* 1996;5:1–11.

54. Kessel L, Watson M: The painful arc syndrome: Clinical classification as a guide to management. *J Bone Joint Surg* 1977;59B:166–172.

55. Petersson CJ, Gentz CF: Ruptures of the supraspinatus tendon: The significance of distally pointing acromioclavicular osteophytes. *Clin Orthop* 1983;174:143–148.

56. Rockwood CA, Lyons FR: Shoulder impingement syndrome: Diagnosis, radiographic evaluation, and treatment with a modified Neer acromioplasty. *J Bone Joint Surg* 1993; 75A:409–424.

57. Aoki M, Ishii S, Usui M: The slope of the acromion and rotator cuff impingement. *Orthop Trans* 1986;10:228.

58. Zuckerman JD, Kummer FJ, Cuomo F, Simon J, Rosenblum S, Katz N: The influence of coracoacromial arch anatomy on rotator cuff tears. *J Shoulder Elbow Surg* 1992;1:4–14.

59. Burns WC II, Whipple TL: Anatomic relationships in the shoulder impingement syndrome. *Clin Orthop* 1993;294:96–102.

60. Jerosch J, Castro WH, Sons HU, Moersler M: Etiology of sub-acromial impingement syndrome: A biomechanical study. *Beitr Orthop Traumatol* 1989;36:411–418.

61. Nasca RJ, Salter EG, Weil CE: Contact areas of the "subacromial" joint, in Bateman JE, Welsh RP (eds): *Surgery of the Shoulder.* Philadelphia, PA, BC Decker, 1984, pp 134–139.

62. Luo ZP, Hsu HC, Morrey BF, An KN: Abstract: Etiologic environment of rotator cuff tears: Intrinsic or extrinsic? *Orthop Trans* 1997; 20:799–800.

63. Flatow EL, Soslowsky LJ, Ticker JB, et al: Excursion of the rotator cuff under the acromion: Patterns of subacromial contact. *Am J Sports Med* 1994;22:779–788.

64. Flatow EL, Coleman WW, Kelkar R, et al: Abstract: The effect of anterior acromioplasty on rotator cuff contact: An experimental and computer simulation. *J Shoulder Elbow Surg* 1995; 4:S53–S54.

65. Caspari RB, Thal R: Arthroscopic subacromial decompression: Technical considerations. *Tech Orthop* 1994;9:102–107.

66. Gohlke F, Daum P, Eulert J: The stabilizing function of the capsule of the glenohumeral joint and the corresponding role of the coracoacromial arch. *J Shoulder Elbow Surg* 1994;3:S24.

67. Lazarus MD, Yung S-W, Sidles JA, Harryman DT II: Anterosuperior humeral displacement: Limitation by the coracoacromial arch. Proceedings of the 62nd Annual Meeting of the American Academy of Orthopaedic Surgeons, Orlando, FL. Rosemont, IL, American Academy of Orthopaedic Surgeons, 1995, p 129.

68. Moorman CT III, Deng X-H, Warren RF, Torzilli PA, Wickiewicz TL: Role of the coracoacromial ligament, coracohumeral veil, and anterior acromiun in stabilizing the glenohumeral joint. Proceedings of the 62nd Annual Meeting of the American Academy of Orthopaedic Surgeons, Orlando, FL. Rosemont, IL, American Academy of Orthopaedic Surgeons, 1995.

69. Wiley AM: Superior humeral dislocation: A complication following decompression and debridement for rotator cuff tears. *Clin Orthop* 1991;263:135–141.

70. Flatow EL, Weinstein DM, Duralde XA, Compito CA, Pollock RG, Bigliani LU: Abstract: Coracoacromial ligament preservation in rotator cuff surgery. *J Shoulder Elbow Surg* 1994;3:S73.

71. Flatow EL, Connor PM, Levine WN, Arroyo JS, Pollock RG, Bigliani LU: Coracoacromial arch reconstruction for anterosuperior subluxation after failed rotator cuff surgery: A preliminary report. *J Shoulder Elbow Surg* 1997;6:228.

72. Inman VT, Saunders JB, Abbott LC: Observations on the function of the shoulder joint. *J Bone Joint Surg* 1944;26:1–30.

73. Turkel SJ, Panio MW, Marshall JL, Girgis FG: Stabilizing mechanisms preventing anterior dislocation of the glenohumeral joint. *J Bone Joint Surg* 1981;63A:1208–1217.

74. Howell SM, Imobersteg AM, Seger DH, Marone PJ: Clarification of the role of the supraspinatus muscle in shoulder function. *J Bone Joint Surg* 1986;68A:398–404.

75. Hughes RE, An K-N: Force analysis of rotator cuff muscles. *Clin Orthop* 1996;330:75–83.

76. Kronberg M, Nemeth G, Brostrom LA: Muscle activity and coordination in the normal shoulder: An electromyographic study. *Clin Orthop* 1990;257:76–85.

77. McCann PD, Wootten ME, Kadaba MP, Bigliani LU: A kinematic and electromyographic study of shoulder rehabilitation exercises. *Clin Orthop* 1993;288:179–188.

78. Sigholm G, Herberts P, Almstrom C, Kadefors R: Electromyographic analysis of shoulder muscle load. *J Orthop Res* 1984;1:379–386.

79. Townsend H, Jobe FW, Pink M, Perry J: Electromyographic analysis of the glenohumeral muscles during a baseball rehabilitation program. *Am J Sports Med* 1991;19:264–272.

80. Otis JC, Jiang CC, Wickiewicz TL, Peterson MG, Warren RF, Santner TJ: Changes in the moment arms of the rotator cuff and deltoid muscles with abduction and rotation. *J Bone Joint Surg* 1994;76A:667–676.

81. Burkhart SS: Reconciling the paradox of rotator cuff repair versus debridement: A unified biomechanical rationale for the treatment of rotator cuff tears. *Arthroscopy* 1994;10:4–19.

82. Thompson WO, Debski RE, Boardman ND III, et al: A biomechanical analysis of rotator cuff deficiency in a cadaveric model. *Am J Sports Med* 1996;24:286–292.

83. Wuelker N, Plitz W, Roetman B: Biomechanical data concerning the shoulder impingement syndrome. *Clin Orthop* 1994;303:242–249.

84. Flatow EL, Kelkar R, Raimondo RA, et al: Abstract: Active and passive restraints against superior humeral translation: The contributions of the rotator cuff, the biceps tendon, and the coracoacromial arch. *J Shoulder Elbow Surg* 1996;5:S111.

85. Glousman R, Jobe F, Tibone J, Moynes D, Antonelli D, Perry J: Dynamic electromyographic analysis of the throwing shoulder with glenohumeral instability. *J Bone Joint Surg* 1988;70A:220–226.

86. Pagnani MJ, Deng XH, Warren RF, Torzilli PA, O'Brien SJ: Role of the long head of the biceps brachii in glenohumeral stability: A biomechanical study in cadavera. *J Shoulder Elbow Surg* 1996;5:255–262.

87. Ting A, Jobe FW, Barto P, Ling B, Moynes D: An EMG analysis of the lateral biceps in shoulders with rotator cuff tears. *Orthop Trans* 1987;11:237.

88. Abbott LC, Saunders JB: Acute traumatic dislocation of the tendon of the long head of the biceps brachii: A report of 6 cases with operative findings. *Surgery* 1939;6:817–840.

89. Burkhead WZ: The biceps tendon, in Rockwood CA, Matsen FA III (eds): *The Shoulder.* Philadelphia, PA, WB Saunders, 1990, pp 791–836.

90. Yamaguchi K, Riew KD, Galantz LM, et al: Biceps function in normal and rotator cuff deficient shoulders: An electromyographic analysis. *Orthop Trans* 1994;18:191.

91. Gilcreest EL: The common syndrome of rupture, dislocation and elongation of the long head of the biceps brachii: An analysis of one hundred cases. *Surg Gynecol Obstet* 1934;58:322–340.

92. Warner JJ, McMahon PJ: The role of the long head of the biceps brachii in superior stability of the glenohumeral joint. *J Bone Joint Surg* 1995;77A:366–372.

ROTATOR CUFF TEARS: PRINCIPLES OF TENDON REPAIR

JONATHAN B. TICKER, MD

JON J.P. WARNER, MD

Neer[1] described four major objectives in surgery for rotator cuff tears: (1) closure of the cuff defect; (2) eliminating the impingement lesions of the coracoacromial arch; (3) preserving the origin of the deltoid muscle; and (4) rehabilitation that prevents postoperative stiffness without disrupting the repair. The principles for techniques of rotator cuff tendon repair and fixation will be discussed in this chapter.

Traditional repairs for supraspinatus tendon tears have included excision of the inflamed bursa, debridement of the edges of the tear, mobilization of the tendon, creation of a trough to the cancellous bone in the sulcus between the articular margin and the greater tuberosity, and closure of the defect with tendon-to-tendon sutures and/or fixation of tendon to bone by means of transosseous sutures.[1–6] A tension-free, water-tight repair was the goal.[7,8] Although these steps have provided good results, recent research and the advent of other methods of repair and of arthroscopy have provided alternatives in the treatment of rotator cuff tears. Arthroscopic techniques have progressed and, in selected cases, they offer the surgeon the ability to repair rotator cuff tears while preserving the deltoid origin.[9–15] Suture anchors have been developed as an alternative to transosseous sutures for rotator cuff tendon repair.[16,17]

SOFT-TISSUE CONSIDERATIONS

Careful management of the soft tissues, especially the bursa and torn tendon edge, is essential to a successful rotator cuff tendon repair. Although resection of bursal tissue is routinely recommended, the literature indicates that the efficacy of this step has not been proved or disproved.[18] Resection of the bursa may serve to enhance exposure of the torn edge of the rotator cuff to facilitate the repair, as well as to remove poten-

tially inflammatory tissue.[19] However, this tissue might provide blood flow and add to the healing response of the repaired tendon, and Bigliani and Rodosky[20] recommend removing only the superficial bursa for this reason. Other surgeons, in order to preserve the gliding function of the bursa, recommend removing only the portion of the bursa that is thickened and scarred or that limits exposure of the rotator cuff tear.[4,21] An additional concern is to clearly differentiate bursa from tendon so that the repair is not compromised by inadvertent removal of tendon with bursa or by use of bursal tissue for the repair instead of tendon.[21]

Preparation of the edge of the rotator cuff has been a routine step in repair of the torn rotator cuff tendon. Early descriptions reported that "freshening the ends" of the torn proximal portion of the tear preceded the repair.[22] McLaughlin[7,8] and DePalma,[4] as well as others, implied that this step in a rotator cuff repair served to remove avascular tissue, and these investigators recommended resection back to a healthy margin.[4,7,8,19,23] Theoretically, a more viable tissue surface would then be available to aid in the healing process.

However, blood flow at the torn edge of rotator cuff tendons has been demonstrated using laser Doppler flowmetry, suggesting that viable tissue is present.[24] Matsen and Arntz[18] stated that the "ratty" border of the tendon should be removed to provide an edge of tissue that is capable of holding a suture. Neer[1] recommended removing only a "thin margin" of the edge of the tear. It would seem that a minimal debridement of the torn rotator cuff tendon edge is necessary at this stage of the procedure to remove "degenerated tissue," and 1 to 2 mm has been suggested.[19,20,25–27]

Early techniques for rotator cuff tendon mobilization included placing tenaculums or forceps on the free edge of the torn rotator cuff.[3,28] Although this procedure may provide the surgeon with a good grip on the tissue, the tendon that is crushed beneath clamps will be considerably less viable, affecting the tissue's ability to hold a suture and to heal. Tenaculums or towel clips may create large holes in the tendon and are not forgiving when used for traction. Placement of traction sutures evenly along the torn edge of the rotator cuff tendon is a superior means of applying tension on the cuff tissue during mobilization and repair.[1] In addition, when passing these sutures through the tendon, taper needles and not cutting needles should be used to minimize both tissue damage and the size of the hole for the suture.

Mobilization of a retracted tendon requires both intra-articular and extra-articular releases. These techniques have been well outlined in the literature.[1,18,20,21]

FIXATION TO BONE

As rotator cuff surgery progressed, it was appreciated that the remaining tissue on the greater tuberosity might be insufficient to support a repair. Although Codman[29] described the repair of the torn rotator cuff to the remaining stump of tendon on the greater tuberosity or through a transosseous mattress suture, most subsequent reports routinely recommended a transosseous suture repair for transversely oriented tears.[1,4–6,18,21,23,26,29–33] In 1931, Wilson[28] recommended repairing the torn edge into a cancellous bone bed. Based on this, McLaughlin[5] in 1944 reported his technique of creating a trough in the sulcus between the greater tuberosity and the humeral articular cartilage. He also noted that the repair could be placed into a trough on the superior humeral articular surface if tension, while repairing the rotator cuff tendon further laterally, was excessive with the arm at the side. Wolfgang[33] noted that the placement of a trough in the articular surface of the humeral head to complete the rotator cuff repair usually led to a worse result. Other recommendations included creating a raw bony surface, which could be quite large, to promote tendon healing.[2,30]

McLaughlin[7,8] believed that "tendon cannot be expected to heal to naked cortical bone or cartilage or to a raveled tendon stump remaining on the humeral tuberosity." It was believed that creating a trough provided a vascular bed for the tendon repair. Furthermore, many investigators have described an area of the supraspinatus with diminished vascularity where rotator cuff pathology usually initiates.[34–36] As a result, most reports recommended placement of a trough in the anatomic neck of the humerus, although without specifying its depth.[18,27,32] Neer[1] recommended placing a shallow 0.5-cm slot where the tendon was detached. Investigators using a dog model demonstrated that a healed rotator cuff repair to a bone trough formed the four zones of a normal tendon insertion at 24 weeks following repair.[37] However, the mean strength of the repaired tendon never achieved that of normal controls.

More recently, the necessity of a trough has been questioned.[20] Bigliani and Rodosky[20] reported that debriding the anatomic neck area with a curette was as effective for tendon-to-bone healing as using a trough. St. Pierre and associates[38] used a goat model to compare the histologic and mechanical properties of rotator cuff tendon attached to a cancellous trough in the bone versus a direct fixation of tendon to the cortical surface using transosseous sutures. In one shoulder of each goat, a 20-mm × 5-mm × 5-mm trough was used at the site of reattachment of the infraspinatus tendon. In the other shoulder of each goat, the insertion site was only debrided of soft tissue. The investigators were unable to demonstrate any difference in load to failure, energy to failure, stiffness, mechanism of failure, or histologic characteristics between the two methods of bone preparation at 6 or 12 weeks following rotator cuff tendon repair. However, they noted that the mechanical properties of both repair techniques remained significantly less than those of the control intact tendon. Therefore, it would seem that a large bone trough is unnecessary for a successful open rotator cuff repair. Furthermore, the creation of a large trough may make repair of a retracted tendon more difficult, because it will increase the distance the tendon must be mobilized to contact bone. This increase may create greater tension on the suture repair.

SUTURE AND THE REPAIR

When performing a primary repair of rotator cuff tendon tears, Gerber and associates[39] suggested that the "ideal repair should have high initial fixation strength, allow minimal gap formation, and maintain mechanical stability until solid healing." In his initial report, Codman[3] used "heavy silk" sutures, a type of material that was used by others.[5,22,23,31] More recent authors have not been as consistent in the type of suture material used for rotator cuff tendon repair. Post[6] recommended size 2-0 sutures of either absorbable or nonabsorbable material, but later recommended heavy nonabsorbable sutures.[19] DePalma[4] used size 1 Vicryl (Ethicon, Sommerville, NJ) or cotton, and Kunkel and Hawkins[32] recommended a size 1 absorbable suture. Nonabsorbable suture material ranging from size 2-0 to size 2 has been recommended by a number of authors.[1,20,21,27]

A single or double loop of suture in a simple fashion has been suggested by some surgeons for the transosseous repair, and a mattress suture technique has been suggested by others.[1,4,27] Although many surgeons[1,5] recommend that sutures be tied laterally on the greater tuberosity, Kunkel and Hawkins[32] recommend a repair with size 1 absorbable suture tied directly over the tendon in a mattress fashion. Suture material that could subsequently cause impingement, such as nonabsorbable suture in the subacromial space, should be avoided.[21] For this reason, Neer[1] has also recommended that side-to-side sutures be buried.

In an attempt to obtain a consensus of opinion, Gerber and associates[39] surveyed 20 active members of the American Shoulder and Elbow Surgeons (ASES) and 10 members of the European Shoulder and Elbow Society. Ninety-six percent of ASES members and 83% of surgeons overall preferred nonabsorbable suture material, with an even distribution for suture size ranging from 0 to 2. In addition, all 30 surgeons used a transosseous method of fixation during rotator cuff repair. These investigators then performed in vitro testing of different suture materials and suture techniques. Although nonabsorbable braided polyester and absorbable braided sutures were found to have similar mechanical properties, the nonabsorbable suture was recommended for clinical use because, unlike an absorbable suture, it can maintain its properties for the duration of tendon-to-bone healing. Monofilament absorbable sutures demonstrated lower tensile strength at failure with greater elongation at loads well below failure. The knots for braided polyester were secure after four simple throws or one surgeon's square knot and two additional simple throws. Furthermore, the suture techniques for grasping the tendon showed considerable variability. For tendon repairs under tension, a modified Mason-Allen locking suture technique demonstrated the least gap formation of the 14 techniques with a high tensile load at failure, while grasping a minimum amount of tendon to reduce strangulation of the tissue (Fig. 10). The mattress suture technique performed in the midrange of the various techniques tested, whereas the simple suture was the weakest. However,

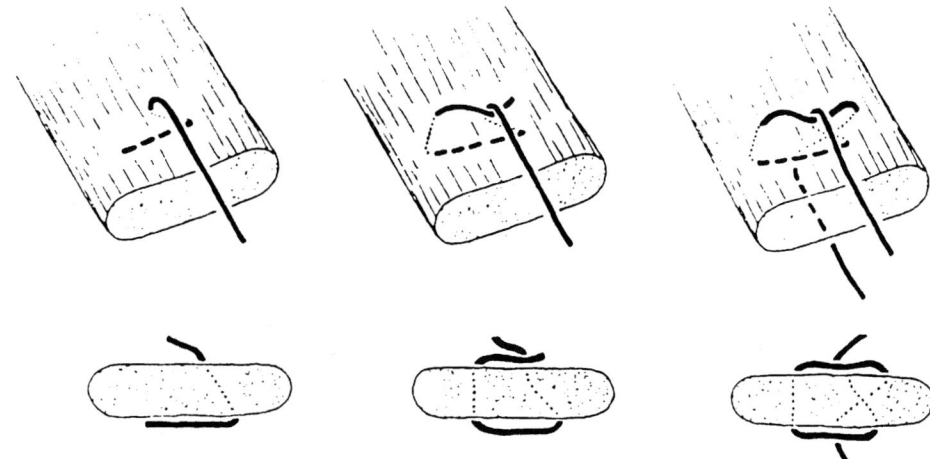

FIGURE 10
Mason-Allen suture repair technique. (Reproduced with permission from Gerber C, Schneeberger AG, Beck M, Schlegel U: Mechanical strength of repairs of the rotator cuff. *J Bone Joint Surg* 1994;76B:371–380.)

these authors noted that a simple suture repair may be an excellent technique for small rotator cuff tears, such as those isolated to the supraspinatus, when the repair is not under tension. A recent study by Burkhart and associates[40] compared the ultimate load to failure for rotator cuff repair with a single mattress suture to repair with two simple sutures. Although both methods of fixation required two bone tunnels, the two simple sutures had a significantly higher ultimate load to failure when compared with the single mattress suture.

Gerber and associates[39] also observed that osteoporotic bone was the "weakest link in the chain," and that augmentation of the cortex of the greater tuberosity sometimes improved fixation. Other investigators have noted that, in a cadaver model, augmentation can improve the initial failure loads of a rotator cuff tendon repair with a mattress suture technique.[41,42] However, intact controls had two to three times the failure load despite these alternative techniques. Therefore, it

remains essential to protect the rotator cuff repair from overloading, and failure, during the early phases of healing.

In my (JJPW) experience, in the optimum transosseous repair configuration, sutures are placed at least 2 cm distal to the tip of the greater tuberosity and are tied over a 1-cm bone bridge (Fig. 11). In biomechanical testing, this configuration has been shown to be two times stronger than sutures tied over a 5-mm bone bridge only 1 cm distal to the tuberosity.[42] The reason for this is that cortical bone thickness increases distal to the tuberosity.

SUTURE ANCHORS

Suture anchor systems were developed to facilitate the repair of soft tissue to bone. A number of pull-out studies were performed to assess the initial fixation strength of these devices, particularly

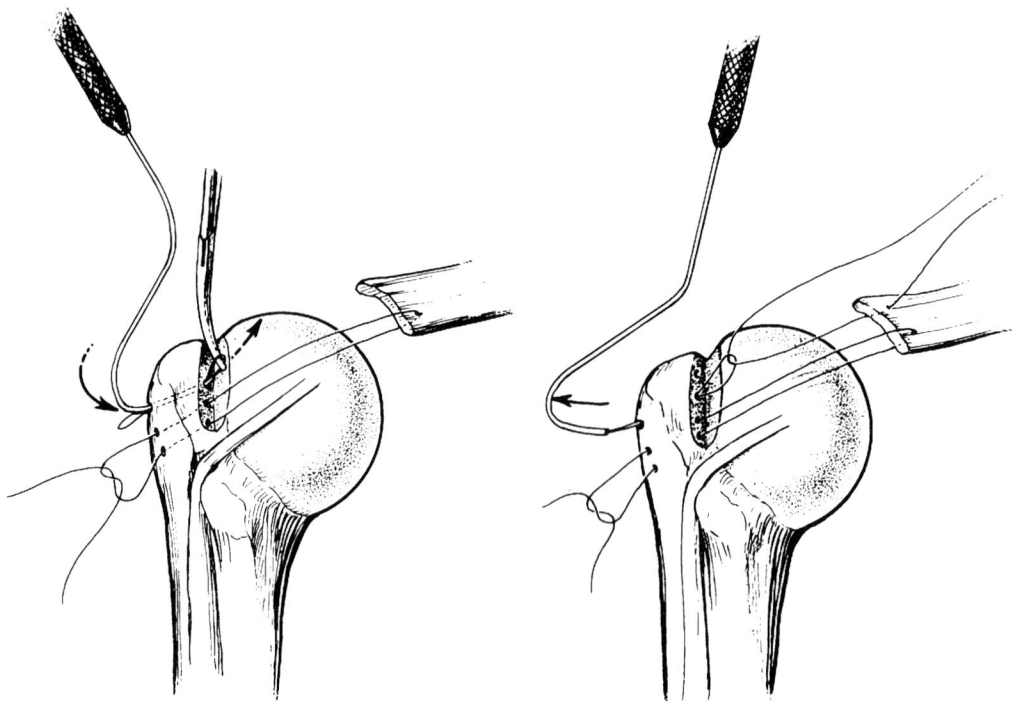

FIGURE 11
Configuration for transosseous repair of rotator cuff tendon. Sutures are tied over a 1 cm bone bridge 2 cm distal to the tip of the greater tuberosity. (Reproduced with permission from Ticker JB, Warner JJP: Single-tendon tears of the rotator cuff. *Orthop Clin North Am* 1997;28:99–116.)

in areas of thin cortical bone or cancellous bone.[43–49] Barber and associates[44–46] used a fresh porcine femur model to study more than 30 different anchors secured with metal wire into thicker cortical bone, thinner cortical bone, and cancellous bone, to test the properties of the anchors and not the suture material. The devices varied and included metallic screw systems, metallic nonscrew systems, plastic systems, and bioabsorbable systems. A few general observations could be made. With very few exceptions, including the bioabsorbable devices, initial loads to failure for the anchors were greater than that for size 2 Ethibond suture (Ethicon, Sommerville, NJ), a nonabsorbable braided polyester. Larger metallic screws had the highest mean load at failure, and nonscrew anchors with larger holes necessary for placement had lower loads at failure in cancellous bone.

Using plastic and metallic nonscrew systems, Carpenter and associates[47] observed that the pull-out strength of suture anchors increased when the load was applied parallel to the bone surface compared with a load applied perpendicular to the bone surface. Testing parallel to the bone surface is more representative of the clinical situation of loading at low angles of arm abduction following rotator cuff repairs. Whereas Carpenter and associates[47] found that the pull-out strength was higher in thicker cortical bone, this was not a consistent finding by Barber and associates.[44,45] Increased pull-out strength of suture anchors in areas of thicker cortical bone would further support a trend to less of a bone trough, or none at all. In an in vivo study using ram femurs, Barber and associates[43] found that the metallic screw and nonscrew anchors failed consistently via suture breakage over the duration of the study. The plastic nonscrew anchor had a lower load at failure initially. At 2 weeks, the load at failure was similar to that for metallic devices, but the mechanism of failure was primarily by suture cut-out from the anchor. At 4 to 12 weeks, the plastic anchor achieved the consistency of the metallic devices with failure by suture breakage. The bioabsorbable device did not achieve a failure load comparable to the other devices until 6 weeks, and the load decreased at the 2- and 4-week marks. It would seem that metallic devices have the potential to maintain mechanical stability during the initial healing phases following rotator cuff repair.

The effectiveness of suture anchor systems was initially demonstrated in the clinical setting for Bankart repairs.[50] Subsequent studies using a cadaver model to test initial fixation strength and a prospective, randomized clinical series both have demonstrated that anchor systems were equally as effective as transosseous sutures along the glenoid rim for Bankart repairs.[48,51] Although early studies of the initial Mitek suture anchor (Mitek Surgical, Inc, Norwood, MA) revealed good fixation strength along the scapular neck, this was not observed when this anchor was placed in the humeral head.[49] Hecker and associates[48] subsequently showed that three anchors used to repair a supraspinatus tear in cadaver shoulders had initial failure strength equal to that of a transosseous repair with three simple sutures. Although there have been reports of the use of suture anchors in open rotator cuff repairs, a prospective, randomized study comparing anchors to transosseous fixation for open rotator cuff repairs is necessary before this technique can be recommended for general use.[9]

The potential for application of suture anchors in rotator cuff surgery may be greatest for arthroscopic techniques. Initial reports of arthroscopic rotator cuff repair have been favorable.[16,17,52,53] Both absorbable and nonabsorbable suture have been used, tied in a mattress fashion directly over the rotator cuff tendon. Pull-out of one anchor has been reported in both of the larger series, although without apparent detrimental effect.[16,17] Indeed, little has been published regarding complications related to suture anchors.[54] Other investigators are developing arthroscopic techniques that are similar to open techniques, using a transosseous method of fixation.[11,55] Based on the information currently available on suture anchors, the observations by Barber and associates[45] should be kept in mind. The effectiveness of a suture anchor depends not only on the initial failure strength, but also on anchor size, anchor composition, suture type, size of the drill hole, and available bone stock. This assumes that other factors are controlled for, such as the technique and skill level of the surgeon.

In our opinion, suture anchor fixation may be acceptable in patients who do not have chronic longstanding tendon tears and associated osteopenia of the greater tuberosity. In a large, long-standing tear in an older individual, there may be disuse osteopenia of the greater tuberosity, which reduces the holding strength of the anchor. In these patients, loss of fixation in the bone is a real possibility if an anchor is used.

SUMMARY

Successful surgical treatment of rotator cuff tendon tears requires attention to technical details. A secure tendon repair depends on careful soft-tissue management and strong fixation to bone during the healing phase. The type of suture, preferably braided nonabsorbable material, and suture technique will affect the repair. Although suture anchors may have a role in rotator cuff repairs, especially if performed arthroscopically, transosseous methods for tendon repair are currently recommended in the majority of cases.

REFERENCES

1. Neer CS II (ed): Cuff tears, biceps lesions, and impingement, in *Shoulder Reconstruction*. Philadelphia, PA, WB Saunders, 1990, pp 41–142.

2. Bosworth DM: An analysis of twenty-eight consecutive cases of incapacitating shoulder lesions, radically explored and repaired. *J Bone Joint Surg* 1940;22:369–392.

3. Codman EA: Complete rupture of the supraspinatus tendon: Operative treatment with report of two successful cases. *Boston Med Surg J* 1911;164:708–710.

4. DePalma AF (ed): Disorders associated with biologic aging of the shoulder: Painful arc syndrome (impingement syndrome), in *Surgery of the Shoulder*, ed 3. Philadelphia, PA, JB Lippincott, 1983, pp 245–265.

5. McLaughlin HL: Lesions of the musculotendinous cuff of the shoulder: I. The exposure and treatment of tears with retraction. *J Bone Joint Surg* 1944;26:31–51.

6. Post M: Injuries to the rotator cuff, in Post M (ed): *The Shoulder: Surgical and Nonsurgical Management*. Philadelphia, PA, Lea & Febiger, 1978, pp 304–328.

7. McLaughlin HL: Rupture of the rotator cuff. *J Bone Joint Surg* 1962;44A:979–983.

8. McLaughlin HL: Repair of major cuff ruptures. *Surg Clin North Am* 1963;43:1535–1540.

9. Armstrong JH: Rotator cuff repair using anchor sutures. *Orthop Trans* 1994;18:312–313.

10. Blevins FT, Warren RF, Cavo C, et al: Arthroscopic-assisted rotator cuff repair: Results using a mini-open deltoid splitting approach. *Arthroscopy* 1996;12:50–59.

11. Flatow EL, Rodosky MW, Compito CA, et al: Abstract: Arthroscopic rotator cuff repair with suture to bone technique: A cadaver study. *Arthroscopy* 1994;10:353–354.

12. Levy HJ, Uribe JW, Delaney LG: Arthroscopic assisted rotator cuff repair: Preliminary results. *Arthroscopy* 1990;6:55–60.

13. Liu SH: Arthroscopically-assisted rotator-cuff repair. *J Bone Joint Surg* 1994;76B:592–595.

14. Liu SH, Baker CL: Arthroscopically assisted rotator cuff repair: Correlation of functional results with integrity of the cuff. *Arthroscopy* 1994;10:54–60.

15. Warner JJP, Altchek DW, Warren RF: Arthroscopic management of rotator cuff tears with emphasis on the throwing athlete. *Op Tech Orthop* 1991;1:235–239.

16. Snyder SJ, Heath DD: Abstract: Arthroscopic repair of rotator cuff tears with miniature suture screw anchors and permanent mattress sutures. *Arthroscopy* 1994;10:345–346.

17. Wolf EM: Arthroscopic rotator cuff repair, in *Book of Abstracts and Instructional Course Outlines*. Rosemont, IL, Arthroscopy Association of North America, 1996, pp 129–132.

18. Matsen FA III, Arntz CT: Rotator cuff tendon failure, in Rockwood CA Jr, Matsen FA III (eds): *The Shoulder*. Philadelphia, PA, WB Saunders, 1990, vol 2, pp 647–677.

19. Post M, Silver R, Singh M: Rotator cuff tear: Diagnosis and treatment. *Clin Orthop* 1983;173:78–91.

20. Bigliani LU, Rodosky MW: Techniques of repair of large rotator cuff tears. *Tech Orthop* 1994;9:133–140.

21. Iannotti JP (ed): *Rotator Cuff Disorders: Evaluation and Treatment.* Park Ridge, IL, American Academy of Orthopaedic Surgeons, 1991.

22. Gray CH: Rupture of the supraspinatus tendon. *Lancet* 1938;1:483–487.

23. Samilson RL, Binder WF: Symptomatic full thickness tears of the rotator cuff: An analysis of 292 shoulders in 276 patients. *Orthop Clin North Am* 1975;6:449–466.

24. Swiontkowski MF, Iannotti JP, Boulas HJ, Esterhai JL: Intraoperative assessment of rotator cuff vascularity using laser Doppler flowmetry, in Post M, Morrey BF, Hawkins RJ (eds): *Surgery of the Shoulder.* St. Louis, MO, Mosby-Year Book, 1990, pp 208–212.

25. Bigliani LU, Cordasco FA, McIlveen SJ, Musso ES: Operative repair of massive rotator cuff tears: Long-term results. *J Shoulder Elbow Surg* 1992;1:120–130.

26. Ellman H, Hanker G, Bayer M: Repair of the rotator cuff: End-result study of factors influencing reconstruction. *J Bone Joint Surg* 1986;68A:1136–1144.

27. Poppen NK: Soft-tissue lesions of the shoulder, in Chapman MW, Madison M (eds): *Operative Orthopaedics,* ed 2. Philadelphia, PA, JB Lippincott, 1993, vol 2, pp 1651–1671.

28. Wilson PD: Complete rupture of the supraspinatus tendon. *JAMA* 1931;96:433–439.

29. Codman EA: Obscure lesions of the shoulder: Rupture of the supraspinatus tendon. *Boston Med Surg J* 1927;196:381–387.

30. Bateman JE: The diagnosis and treatment of ruptures of the rotator cuff. *Surg Clin North Am* 1963;43:1523–1530.

31. Davis TW, Sullivan JF: Rupture of the supraspinatus tendon. *Ann Surg* 1937;106:1059–1069.

32. Kunkel SS, Hawkins RJ: Rotator cuff repair utilizing a trough in bone, in Paulos LE, Tibone JE (eds): *Operative Techniques in Shoulder Surgery.* Gaithersburg, MD, Aspen Publishers, 1991, pp 149–154.

33. Wolfgang GL: Surgical repair of tears of the rotator cuff of the shoulder: Factors influencing the result. *J Bone Joint Surg* 1974;56A:14–26.

34. Moseley HF, Goldie I: The arterial pattern of the rotator cuff of the shoulder. *J Bone Joint Surg* 1963;45B:780–789.

35. Rathbun JB, Macnab I: The microvascular pattern of the rotator cuff. *J Bone Joint Surg* 1970;52B:540–553.

36. Rothman RH, Parke WW: The vascular anatomy of the rotator cuff. *Clin Orthop* 1965;41:176–186.

37. Miyahara H, Takagishi K, Arita C, Arai K, Hotokebuchi T, Sugioka Y: A morphologic and biomechanical study on the healing of the repaired rotator cuff insertion in dogs: A preliminary report, in Post M, Morrey BF, Hawkins RJ (eds): *Surgery of the Shoulder.* St. Louis, MO, Mosby-Year Book, 1990, pp 224–227.

38. St. Pierre P, Olson EJ, Elliott JJ, O'Hair KC, McKinney LA, Ryan J: Tendon-healing to cortical bone compared with healing to a cancellous trough: A biomechanical and histological evaluation in goats. *J Bone Joint Surg* 1995;77A:1858–1866.

39. Gerber C, Schneeberger AG, Beck M, Schlegel U: Mechanical strength of repairs of the rotator cuff. *J Bone Joint Surg* 1994;76B:371–380.

40. Burkhart SS, Fischer SP, Nottage WM, et al: Abstract: Tissue fixation security in transosseous rotator cuff repairs: A mechanical comparison of simple versus mattress sutures, in *Book of Abstracts and Instructional Course Outlines.* Rosemont, IL, Arthroscopy Association of North America, 1996, p 65.

41. France EP, Paulos LE, Harner CD, Straight CB: Biomechanical evaluation of rotator cuff fixation methods. *Am J Sports Med* 1989;17:176–181.

42. Caldwell GL, Warner JJP, Miller MD, Boardman D, Towers J, Debski R: Strength of fixation with transosseous sutures in rotator cuff repair. *J Bone Joint Surg* 1997;79A:1064–1068.

43. Barber FA, Cawley P, Prudich JF: Suture anchor failure strength: An in vivo study. *Arthroscopy* 1993;9:647–652.

44. Barber FA, Herbert MA, Click JN: The ultimate strength of suture anchors. *Arthroscopy* 1995;11:21–28.

45. Barber FA, Herbert MA, Click JN: Suture anchor strength revisited. *Arthroscopy* 1996;12:32–38.

46. Barber FA, Herbert MA, Click JN: Recent suture anchor developments, in *Book of Abstracts and Instructional Course Outlines*. Rosemont, IL, Arthroscopy Association of North America, 1996, pp 82–83.

47. Carpenter JE, Fish DN, Huston LJ, Goldstein SA: Pull-out strength of five suture anchors. *Arthroscopy* 1993;9:109–113.

48. Hecker AT, Shea M, Hayhurst JO, Myers ER, Meeks LW, Hayes WC: Pull-out strength of suture anchors for rotator cuff and Bankart lesion repairs. *Am J Sports Med* 1993;21:874–879.

49. Paulos LE, France EP, Harner CD: Biomechanical evaluation of rotator cuff fixation methods, in Post M, Morrey BF, Hawkins RJ (eds): *Surgery of the Shoulder*. St. Louis, MO, Mosby-Year Book, 1990, pp 220–223.

50. Richmond JC, Donaldson WR, Fu F, Harner CD: Modification of the Bankart reconstruction with a suture anchor: Report of a new technique. *Am J Sports Med* 1991;19:343–346.

51. Norlin R: Use of Mitek anchoring for Bankart repair: A comparative, randomized, prospective study with traditional bone sutures. *J Shoulder Elbow Surg* 1994;3:381–385.

52. Snyder SJ, Bachner EJ: Abstract: Arthroscopic fixation of rotator cuff tears: A preliminary report. *Arthroscopy* 1993;9:342.

53. Tippett JW: Abstract: Arthroscopic rotator cuff repairs, in *Book of Abstracts and Instructional Course Outlines*. Rosemont, IL, Arthroscopy Association of North America, 1996, p 66.

54. Ticker JB, Lippe RJ, Barkin DE, Carroll MP: Infected suture anchors in the shoulder: A case report. *Arthroscopy* 1996;12:613–615.

55. Burkhart SS. Arthroscopic drill-hook rotator cuff repair through bone tunnels: A problem-solution approach, in *Book of Abstracts and Instructional Course Outlines*. Rosemont, IL, Arthroscopy Association of North America, 1996, pp 133–145.

ARTHROSCOPIC ACROMIOPLASTY AND ARTHROSCOPIC DISTAL CLAVICLE RESECTION, MINI-OPEN ROTATOR CUFF REPAIR: INDICATIONS, TECHNIQUES, AND OUTCOME

CHARLES W. HARTZOG, JR, MD, FELIX H. SAVOIE, III, MD, LARRY D. FIELD, MD

INTRODUCTION

The advent of arthroscopy has added to the understanding and management of disorders of the shoulder. The arthroscope is a valuable tool that has allowed for improvements not only in the accurate diagnosis of shoulder pathology but in its effective management as well. This chapter will focus primarily on arthroscopy and arthroscopic assisted management of impingement syndrome, acromioclavicular arthritis, and rotator cuff tears.

IMPINGEMENT SYNDROME

The etiology of rotator cuff pathology has been attributed to both extrinsic and intrinsic factors. Primary extrinsic factors include acromial shape, os acromiale, acromioclavicular (AC) joint pathology, hypertrophy of the coracoacromial ligament, and chronic synovitis of the subacromial bursa.[1-3] Secondary extrinsic factors include instability, posterior capsular tightness, and abnormal muscular or neurogenic control of the rotator cuff.[1,4-6] Intrinsic causes including overuse and insufficient blood supply have been proposed by Nirschl,[7] and Rathbun and Macnab.[8]

Impingement syndrome and its coincident progression of rotator cuff disease has been described by Neer,[9,10] who divided rotator cuff pathology into three distinct stages, recognizing that this pathology is a continuum; stage I consists of reversible changes of edema and hemorrhage within the rotator cuff tendons; stage II consists of irreversible changes of fibrosis and tendinitis; and stage III pathology is marked by disruption and tearing of the rotator cuff tendons. Recently,

Jobe[11] determined instability to be a cause of impingement-like symptoms in athletes. Currently, impingement is believed to be multifactorial, with age (vascular changes, tendon degeneration), mechanical considerations (spurs, dysvascularity), and instability contributing to varying degrees.

The initial evaluation of the patient with shoulder pain is extremely important. Misdiagnosis has been reported to be a leading cause of failure of arthroscopic acromioplasty.[12-15] A thorough history, physical examination, and radiographic studies as indicated should be performed. Specific entities that must be excluded are cervical radiculopathy/spondylosis, acromioclavicular arthritis, glenohumeral arthritis, glenohumeral instability, suprascapular nerve entrapment, thoracic outlet syndrome, ulnar nerve entrapment, labral tears, and adhesive capsulitis.

Patient Presentation

The typical patient with impingement syndrome usually presents with pain on overhead activities along with diminished function above shoulder level. Nocturnal pain is often present. There often is no history of injury, and the pain is usually progressive. Classic physical examination findings include a positive impingement sign in frontal flexion of 140°, a secondary impingement sign (pain/popping on internal and external rotation with the arm forward flexed), subacromial crepitation, and a positive impingement test (diminution of pain with subacromial injection). Weakness of the supraspinatus and external rotators may also be noted. Tests for instability, such as the apprehension, relocation, and load and shift tests, should always be performed. In isolated impingement syndrome resulting from subacromial outlet narrowing, these tests will be negative.

Standard radiographs, including anteroposterior (AP), axillary lateral, and the "outlet view" described by Morrison and Bigliani[16] (Fig. 12), should be taken. Radiographic findings of patients with rotator cuff pathology may include acromial spurring, inferior AC osteophytes, sclerosis of either the greater tuberosity or the anterior acromion, superior migration of the humeral head, or calcification of the supraspinatus tendon. Further delineation of the extent of rotator cuff pathology can be obtained by arthrogram or magnetic resonance imaging (MRI).

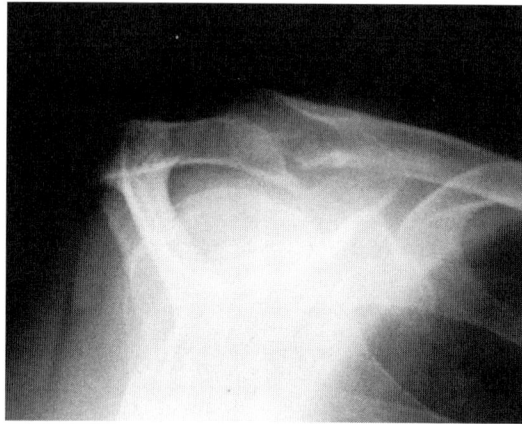

FIGURE 12
"Outlet view" as described by Morrison and Bigliani.[16] Note type III (hooked) acromial morphology with elongated anterior acromial spur formation.

Management

Once a diagnosis of impingement syndrome has been established, all patients should undergo a trial of nonsurgical therapy. This protocol should include behavior modification to control painful motions and stepwise progression of a physical therapy program directed at stretching and strengthening of the rotator cuff musculature, the deltoid, and the periscapular stabilizers. All therapy initially should be performed below 90° of flexion to improve the effectiveness of the depressors of the humeral head and should be accompanied by the application of ice after therapy

sessions to minimize discomfort. Nonsteroidal anti-inflammatory medications, as well as the judicious use of subacromial cortisone injections and oral corticosteroids, should be employed.

Neer's[9] original description of an anterior acromioplasty involves detachment of a small segment of the deltoid origin anteriorly to provide access to the subacromial space. He describes removal of a wedge-shaped portion of bone from the anterior acromion and states this removed segment of bone should be at least 9 mm anteriorly and tapered posteriorly for a distance of 2 cm. This technique of open acromioplasty has maintained a high degree of success with multiple authors reporting patient satisfaction from 86% to 95%.[17–19] The technique of arthroscopic acromioplasty was initially described by Ellman[20] in 1987. Since then, multiple authors have reported results comparable to those of open acromioplasty.[14,15,21–31]

Regardless of the technique used, the objectives of subacromial decompression should always be the same. Those primary objectives are to debride the hypertrophic bursa, to release the coracoacromial ligament, to resect the undersurface of the anterior acromion producing a smooth acromial undersurface, and to excise any AC osteophytes to the same level as the anterior acromion.[12,15,24,32–34]

Difficulties encountered when performing arthroscopic subacromial decompression include the control of bleeding, the knowledge of how much bone to resect, and the proper contouring of the acromial undersurface.[32–35] The shoulder does not lend itself to tourniquet control of hemorrhage, and the subacromial space lacks a synovial lining to act as a fluid-restricting barrier.[36,37] These difficulties can, however, be overcome.

A properly performed arthroscopic subacromial decompression has many advantages. This procedure requires less dissection, has less morbidity, and is more cosmetic than the comparable open procedure. Because the deltoid origin is not formally released, there is less postoperative discomfort. Also, an intact deltoid allows for a more aggressive rehabilitation protocol with immediate active range of motion, shortening recovery time.

Altchek and associates[14] have reported that 89% of their patients returned to work within 1 week of the procedure. Arthroscopic acromioplasty is performed on an outpatient basis, decreasing hospital costs. The arthroscope allows for direct visualization of the subacromial space with confirmation of the findings of impingement, detection of any AC joint pathology, and evaluation of rotator cuff tears if open surgery is planned.[14,24,38–40]

An additional advantage of the arthroscopic approach is that it provides direct visualization and inspection of the glenohumeral joint for detection and treatment of intra-articular pathology. Paulos and Franklin[15] have documented compromised clinical results when treatment of glenohumeral pathology was omitted. Several authors have documented the increased frequency of associated pathology in patients with impingement syndrome or full-thickness rotator cuff tears.[14,22,39,40] Specific glenohumeral lesions noted have included synovitis, labral tears, abnormalities of the articular cartilage (including glenoid and humeral head arthritic changes), biceps tendon tears, instability, loose bodies, and adhesive capsulitis.[39,40]

ACROMIOCLAVICULAR ARTHRITIS

AC joint pathology can exist as an isolated entity or as part of a global shoulder condition. The first step in its proper treatment is to make a correct and accurate diagnosis using history, physical examination, and proper radiographic studies.

Patients with isolated AC disease will often present with anterior-superior shoulder pain that is exacerbated by activity. This pain may often radiate to the base of the neck or to the trapezius, leading to spasm, and may often be worse at night. A specific history of trauma may indicate an acute or chronic AC separation. Repetitive microtrauma may also lead to isolated AC disease such as that seen in weight lifters and gymnasts.

Patients who present with AC disease are most often tender to palpation directly over the AC joint. Pain localized to the AC joint may also be elicited with specific provocative maneuvers, such as horizontal adduction of the involved extremity, or with extremes of internal rotation of the involved arm. They may also exhibit a positive "resisted AC compression test," which is pain elicited by resistance to adduction torque with the arm at 90° forward flexion in neutral adduction/abduction and neutral rotation. These patients may exhibit a cosmetic asymmetry of the AC joints. AC crepitus may also be palpable at the area of involvement. Injection of 1% lidocaine into the AC joint may be diagnostic of pathology if pain on provocative testing is subsequently eliminated. This injection may also be therapeutic if steroids are used.

Appropriate radiographs include the standard shoulder series previously mentioned. In addition, a 10° to 15° cephalic tilt AP view using soft-tissue technique can sometimes be helpful (Fig. 13). With this reduced penetration technique, the AC joint can be more accurately visualized and there is no superimposition of the posterior aspect of the acromion. Radiographic findings may include osteolysis of the distal clavicle with cystic formation and arthritic changes, such as clavicular or acromial osteophytes, narrowing of the joint space, and subchondral cysts. With a history of trauma, there may be evidence of inferior displacement of the acromion as compared to the contralateral shoulder.

Additional radiographic studies may be useful in making the diagnosis. Technetium bone scan may show increased uptake at the area of the

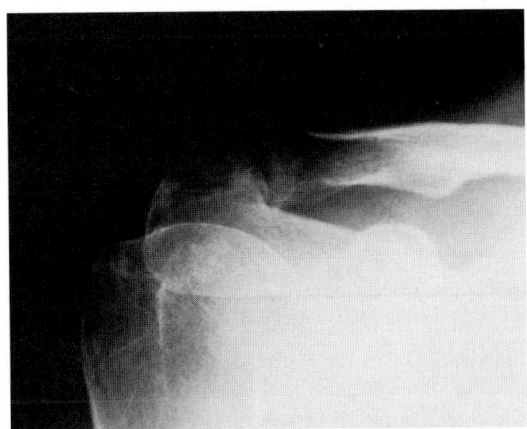

FIGURE 13
This 15° cephalic tile anteroposterior view using soft-tissue technique illustrates the presence of acromioclavicular arthritis.

AC joint.[41] Computed tomography (CT) scans may show narrowing of the joint space, subchondral cysts, or clavicular resorption, but are rarely necessary.[42] These changes may also be evident on MRI performed for other pathologic entities about the shoulder.

Once a diagnosis of AC disease has been made, an appropriate nonsurgical therapeutic program should be instituted. A majority of these patients should improve with a conservative program, including nonsteroidal anti-inflammatory medications, heat, avoidance of painful activities, appropriate physical therapy, and the judicious use of AC steroid injections.

Since its introduction independently by Mumford[43] and Gurd,[44] open distal clavicle resection has been used to treat a variety of AC entities. These have included posttraumatic arthritis, idiopathic osteolysis or osteoarthritis, inflammatory arthritis, distal clavicle fractures, AC separations, and synovial chondromatosis.[45–48] The initial descriptions of the technique of distal clavicle excision included splitting the fascia overlying the acromioclavicular joint with exposure of the distal 2 to 2.5 cm of clavicle for excision.[43,44] Many have obtained reliable results using this technique.[43–45,47,49]

Disadvantages of open distal clavicle excision also have been reported. These include lack of cosmesis of the surgical incision,[45] abutment of the distal clavicle on the acromion secondary to instability,[42,46,49–52] and postoperative shoulder weakness.[49,53,54]

The initial descriptions of arthroscopic distal clavicle resection were given by Ellman[20] in 1987 and Esch and associates[55] in 1988. Since then many authors have reported results equivalent to those of open distal clavicle resection.[41,42,50,51,56–58]

The arthroscopic technique of distal clavicle resection has many advantages. The avoidance of detachment of the trapezius insertion and the deltoid origin allows rapid return to function and should result in less long-term weakness.[41,51,56–58] Cosmesis is much improved. The procedure is performed on an outpatient basis, reducing hospital costs. The arthroscopic technique also allows for maintenance of the integrity of the superior AC capsule, as well as the superior AC ligaments.[51,57,58] The superior and inferior AC ligaments have been proven to be the primary restraints to anterior and posterior displacement of the distal clavicle.[59,60] The preservation of these superior ligaments eliminates the postoperative instability reported after open resection.[49–51,56]

DISORDERS OF THE ROTATOR CUFF

The initial diagnosis of rotator cuff tear is obtained by history, physical examination, and appropriate imaging studies. The clinical presentation of these patients is similar to those with impingement syndrome. Complaints of weakness may be more pronounced with larger tears. There may often be a history of trauma as an initiating event to these symptoms.

Physical examination findings may include profound supraspinatus weakness with testing of the arm at 90° abduction in the plane of the scapula. Strength of the external rotators may also be diminished with larger rotator cuff tears. Subscapularis tears may be identified by a positive lift-off test, or the inability to lift the hand off the back in the internally rotated position.

The findings noted on standard radiographs were previously described. Once the diagnosis of rotator cuff tear has been established, a nonsurgical protocol, which is similar to that used in patients with impingement syndrome, can be considered in some patients. Patients who have acute large tears that occur as a result of single-event trauma and who demonstrate significant weakness should be considered for early rotator cuff repair. For those patients who continue to be symptomatic despite an appropriate conservative program, surgical intervention is indicated. Surgical options include decompression with debridement of the rotator cuff or decompression combined with rotator cuff repair. Despite acceptable results of debridement and decompression alone in select cases,[20,61–63] rotator cuff repair has proven superior for the majority of patients.[12,64,65] Compared to debridement and decompression alone, repair of the rotator cuff provides improved function and strength of the rotator cuff, prevents extension of the tear with possible long-term pain and weakness, and allows complete repair in one surgical setting.[66]

Advances in arthroscopic technique now allow successful subacromial decompression and distal clavicle resection. Advances have also been made in techniques of rotator cuff repair. Surgical options for rotator cuff repair now include arthroscopic cuff repair, arthroscopic assisted/mini-open cuff repair or formal open rotator cuff repair. Most authors have reported good overall results from open rotator cuff repair, combined with subacromial decompression.[67–71] Pain relief has been documented in 71% to 100% of patients and improved function in 72% to 82% of patients.[72] Recent reports of arthroscopically assisted rotator cuff repair have indicated results equivalent to or superior to those of open rotator cuff repair.[66,72–75]

There are many advantages to the use of arthroscopy in the treatment of full-thickness rotator cuff tears. In addition to those previously mentioned, the arthroscope allows direct visualization of the tear for evaluation and planning of its repair via either arthroscopic or open techniques. We perform arthroscopy before every rotator cuff repair. Acromioplasty and distal clavicle resection are performed arthroscopically, followed by an arthroscopic evaluation of the rotator cuff tear.

Several factors should be considered when deciding the method of repair of a particular rotator cuff tear. Important determinants in the success of arthroscopic and arthroscopic assisted techniques include size and location of the tear, retraction of the tear, excursion of the remaining tendon, and quality of both bone and soft tissues.[75,76] Regardless of repair technique, surgical goals are to improve function, decrease pain, and to prevent subsequent extension of the rotator cuff tear.

INDICATIONS

ARTHROSCOPIC ACROMIOPLASTY

The indications for arthroscopic acromioplasty are identical to those for open subacromial decompression.[24,40] The primary indication includes advanced stage II and stage III rotator cuff disease that has not responded to appropriate nonsurgical treatment over a period of at least 6 months. Other specific diagnostic indications include calcific tendinitis, a prominent greater tuberosity (such as after a fracture), and failed rotator cuff repair with an intact deltoid.[32,39,63]

The role of arthroscopy in the treatment of full-thickness rotator cuff tears has been somewhat controversial. Neviaser in 1987 (personal communication) and Brems[77] in 1988 found the arthroscope to be of little value in treating full-thickness rotator cuff tears. The early results of arthroscopic subacromial decompression and debridement as a treatment for full-thickness rotator cuff tears were promising.[20,63] With a 2-year follow-up, Levy and associates[63] reported 84% good and excellent results using the UCLA (University of California at Los Angeles) shoulder rating scale in their initial report of 25 patients with full-thickness rotator cuff tears treated in this manner. They reported that smaller tears seemed to do better than larger tears, although all patients improved. They concluded that this technique should be considered in selected patients with full-thickness rotator cuff tears.

Early enthusiasm over debridement and decompression alone for treatment of full-thickness rotator cuff tears has waned. In 1994, Zvijac and associates[78] reported on the 25 patients originally described by Levy and associates.[63] Findings with an additional 2-year follow-up included 68% good and excellent results compared to the previous 84%, indicating deterioration of these results over time. Other authors have also shown the inadequacy of this method of treating full-thickness rotator cuff tears.[12,64,65] Montgomery and associates[65] detailed the results of 88 chronic full-thickness rotator cuff tears treated by either open surgical tendon repair with anterior acromioplasty or arthroscopic debridement and subacromial decompression. With evaluation by the UCLA shoulder rating scale at 2- to 5-years' follow-up, the results of the open surgical repair group were significantly better than those of the debridement and decompression group. We therefore recommend surgical repair of all full-thickness rotator cuff tears whenever possible, either by arthroscopic or open techniques.

Contraindications to arthroscopic acromioplasty are quite few. The only absolute contraindication is acute cellulitis or other soft-tissue infection about the shoulder. Relative contraindications include uncontrolled hypertension and bleeding disorders.[24,36]

ARTHROSCOPIC DISTAL CLAVICLE RESECTION

The indications for arthroscopic distal clavicle resection are similar to those for open distal clavicle resection. Pain secondary to acromioclavicular (AC) joint pathology that has not been relieved by at least 4 to 6 months of appropriate nonsurgical therapy should be addressed with surgical intervention. Specific lesions of the AC joint may be secondary to osteolysis or arthritis. Osteolysis may be caused by inflammatory arthritis, such as rheumatoid arthritis, by hyperparathyroidism, or by repetitive microtrauma. Although acromioclavicular arthritis may occur after significant trauma, including grade II AC separations and type III distal clavicle intra-articular fractures, it is most often idiopathic in nature.

Although open distal clavicle excision has been recommended in the past for symptomatic AC dislocation,[46] some studies have shown poor results for arthroscopic distal clavicle resection. Bigliani and associates[56] in 1993 found only 37% satisfactory results in those patients who had arthroscopic distal clavicle resection for grade II AC separations. In 1995, Flatow and associates[51] found similarly poor results. Of those patients who had arthroscopic distal clavicle resection for symptomatic grade II AC separation or for painful hypermobility of the AC joint, only 58% achieved satisfactory results.

Poor results in these two studies were attributed to preexisting instability. Without ligamentous continuity of the AC joint, the posterior aspect of the distal clavicle was allowed to abut the acromion or scapular spine when the arm was taken through a range of motion. For this reason, Flatow and associates[51] recommended not only distal clavicle resection, but also a ligamentous reconstruction of the AC joint in these patients.

As previously stated, AC joint pathology may exist as an isolated entity or as part of a more global syndrome about the shoulder. It is extremely important to diagnose AC joint disease in these patients. Neer[9] in 1972 recognized that undiagnosed AC arthritis was a common cause of poor surgical outcome following shoulder surgery performed for other conditions. The history and physical examination is very important in these individuals because previous studies have proven that symptoms of AC disease do not necessarily correlate with the radiographic appearance of the AC joint.[79,80] Watson[81] in 1978 and Neviaser and associates[82] in 1982 recommended routine AC joint resection as part of the subacromial decompression.

ROTATOR CUFF REPAIR

Indications for surgical treatment of rotator cuff tears are similar to those for impingement. These include continued pain and functional disability despite appropriate nonsurgical measures for 3 to 6 months.[66,72,73] Although not mandatory, preoperative documentation by arthrogram or MRI is often valuable. Full-thickness rotator cuff tears in patients younger than 50 years of age deserve special consideration. We feel it is appropriate to perform an arthrogram or MRI acutely in these patients. A positive imaging study for a rotator cuff tear in this patient population is an indication for surgical repair. Those patients with a negative study should be treated nonsurgically as previously described. We believe all symptomatic tears that are not responsive to nonsurgical measures and are amenable to repair should be repaired. The decision then becomes which method of repair is most appropriate.

Arthroscopic Rotator Cuff Repair

Arthroscopic rotator cuff repair techniques remain developmental. There currently are no absolute indications. Early results and limitations of this technique are in the process of being defined. For those surgeons skilled in arthroscopy, however, this certainly seems to be a viable alternative to standard open rotator cuff repair. Tears that we have found amenable to arthroscopic repair include small and moderate sized tears (up to 3 cm) in which there is adequate excursion of the tendon to allow apposition to the greater tuberosity. Bone and tendon quality must also be adequate to allow arthroscopic fixation. If the combination of these factors does not allow a secure, tension-free repair, then open techniques should be used.[76]

Mini-Open Rotator Cuff Repair

Indications for mini-open rotator cuff repair are similar to those for the arthroscopic technique. In 1994, Paulos and Kody[75] noted this technique to be appropriate in acute tears that easily could be mobilized. They also stated that regardless of the size of the tear, retraction should not exceed 2 cm. Baker and Liu[72,73] have defined similar indications. They feel the arthroscopic assisted approach is appropriate for full-thickness tears of small and moderate sizes. They also state that tears up to 5 cm can be repaired using this technique, as long as only minimal to moderate (less than 2 cm) retraction exists.[72] The extended mini-open approach may be used for larger tears. This involves proximal extension of the standard mini-open incision with release of the deltoid origin from the anterior margin of the acromion.

TECHNIQUES

ARTHROSCOPIC ACROMIOPLASTY

The objectives of open acromioplasty and arthroscopic acromioplasty are the same; it is only the techniques by which these objectives are met that differ. When performing arthroscopic acromioplasty, proper orientation and visualization are essential. Therefore, a thorough bursectomy is required to visualize the bursal side of the cuff and orient the acromion within the subacromial space. Maintenance of adequate distention, hemostasis, and traction are required for completion of the procedure.[20,38]

The control of bleeding within the subacromial space can be a challenge. Tips for the maintenance of hemostasis include discontinuing nonsteroidal anti-inflammatory medications at least

1 week before the surgical procedure, placing 1 cc of epinephrine (1 to 1,000 concentration) in each 3-liter bag of irrigant, and maintaining systolic blood pressure in the 90 to 100 mm Hg range.[12,32,33] Additional methods to help control bleeding include placement of a dedicated inflow cannula anteriorly, or the use of a pump, and resection of the bony insertion of the coracoacromial ligament rather than the ligament itself in order to avoid the acromial branch of the thoracoacromial artery.[26]

Arthroscopic acromioplasty requires certain standard equipment. A suction-type bean bag and an upper extremity traction tower are needed to maintain the patient in the lateral decubitus position with the arm positioned appropriately. These elements are not needed for the beach chair position. A standard 30° arthroscope with monitor and a gravity or pump irrigation system are needed. Specialized instruments include a motorized arthroscopic burr, a synovial resector, and, possibly, an electrocautery.

Arthroscopic acromioplasty can be performed in either the lateral decubitus or beach chair position (Fig. 14). The general techniques of decompression are similar for both positions. Most early technical descriptions of arthroscopic subacromial decompression are essentially modifications of Ellman's[20] original technique.

Ellman Technique

Ellman's[20] technique involves placing the patient in the lateral decubitus position with the involved extremity suspended with 10 to 15 lb of traction in a 15° to 20° abducted position and slight forward flexion. The bony landmarks and portal sites are marked with a marking pen. The glenohumeral joint is distended with approximately 30 cc of normal saline solution. A standard posterior portal is established. Diagnostic glenohumeral arthroscopy is then performed, when any pathologic lesion is treated.

The instruments are then repositioned within the subacromial space. The posterior portal is used for fluid inflow. An accessory posterolateral portal is used for introduction of the arthroscope into the subacromial space. Instrumentation is carried out through an anterolateral portal approximately 2 to 3 cm distal to the anterior margin of the acromion. The anterolateral edge of the acromion and the acromioclavicular joint are marked with 22-gauge needles. From the anterolateral portal, a subtotal bursectomy is then carried out with a full radius resector. The coracoacromial ligament is released from its attachment to the acromion with an electrocautery tip. Initially this procedure required the use of distilled water; however, these tips are now plastic coated and can be used in the presence of normal saline solution.

After release of the coracoacromial ligament, electrocautery is used to morcellize the soft tissue underneath the acromion. A synovial resector is used to debride this undersurface, completely exposing the underneath surface of the acromion. A 4.5-mm burr is then used for bony excision. Ellman[20] proposed the use of a deepening hole, using the burr as a means of accurate determination of the depth of bony excision. This 3-mm hole is placed into the anterior acromion and then extended into a trough over the anterior 2 cm of the acromion. It is then widened successively throughout the entire width of the acromion. This process is then repeated until the appropriate depth of acromial resection is achieved. The anterior edge of the acromion is then tapered and recessed a distance of 6 to 8 mm, until it is posterior to the anterior border of the distal clavicle. The acromioclavicular joint should then be inspected and any inferior osteophytes excised. Portals are closed with nylon sutures to complete the procedure.

Various authors have modified this technique.[14,15,24,83] Typical modifications include the use of the standard posterior portal for visualization within the subacromial space. A dedicated inflow is positioned through the anterior portal. The lateral portal typically is used for bursectomy, release of the coracoacromial ligament, and anterior acromioplasty. The coracoacromial ligament typically is released with either electrocautery or with an arthroscopic burr used to undermine the bony insertion of the ligament. Our preferred technique is a modification of that described by Caspari and Thal.[32]

Caspari Technique

Experienced anesthesia personnel administer interscalene block anesthesia with the patient in the holding area. Once the patient is taken into the operating room, general endotracheal anesthesia may also be administered. An examination of both shoulders under anesthesia is then carried

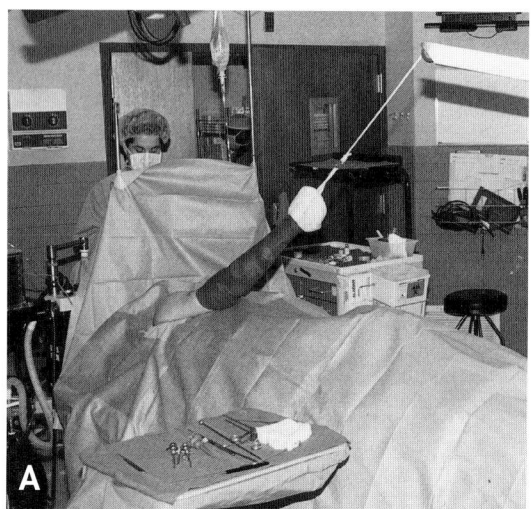
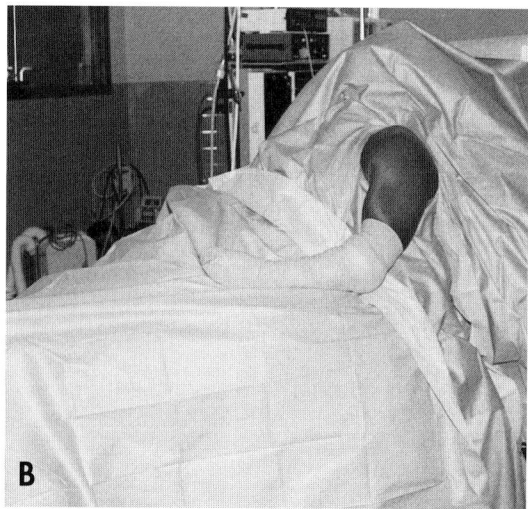

FIGURE 14
A, Demonstration of the lateral decubitus position after standard orthopaedic preparation and drape. **B,** Demonstration of the beach chair position after standard orthopaedic preparation and drape.

out with the patient in the supine position. Particular attention is directed toward the diagnosis of subtle instability, which may not have been noted in the preoperative examination.

Upon completion of the examination under anesthesia, the patient is placed in the lateral decubitus position, all bony prominences are well padded, and the head is supported by a foam bolster to prevent any areas of undue pressure or neurologic injury. The upper torso is tilted posteriorly approximately 30° to maintain the glenohumeral joint in a horizontal orientation. This position is maintained with use of a suction-type bean bag. The patient is taped to the bed for added security. The involved shoulder is prepped and draped in typical orthopaedic fashion. The upper extremity is then suspended at an angle of approximately 45° abduction and 10° to 15° forward flexion with 5 to 10 lbs of skin traction. We are careful to avoid undue pressure at the wrist or elbow (Outline 1).

A standard posterior portal is established at the level of the equator of the glenohumeral joint. Then a 4.5-mm cannula with blunt trocar is inserted into the glenohumeral joint directed toward the coracoid process anteriorly. After confirming that the scope is within the glenohumeral joint, lactated Ringer's solution is used to distend the joint through the side port of the arthroscopic bridge. Diagnostic arthroscopy of the glenohumeral joint is then carried out. It includes inspection of both the glenoid and humeral head articular surfaces; the biceps tendon; superior, middle, and inferior glenohumeral ligaments; the labrum; and the articular surface of the rotator cuff, including the subscapularis tendon.

Upon completion of diagnostic and therapeutic glenohumeral arthroscopy, subacromial bursoscopy is performed. The 4.5-mm arthroscopic cannula with blunt trocar is inserted through the standard posterior portal and directed superiorly into the subacromial space. It is swept from medial to lateral to break up subacromial adhesions. The coracoacromial ligament can be palpated with this blunt trocar. The trocar is then pushed through a previously established anterior portal, just lateral to the coracoacromial ligament. From

OUTLINE 1

STEPS OF ARTHROSCOPIC ACROMIOPLASTY

1. Lateral decubitus position with patient tilted back 30°
2. Diagnostic glenohumeral arthroscopy with treatment of intra-articular lesions
3. Subacromial bursoscopy
4. Posterior visualization portal
5. Anterior inflow portal
6. Establish lateral instrumentation portal 3 cm from anterolateral edge of acromion
7. Perform subtotal bursectomy with 4.5-mm synovial resector blade
8. Release coracoacromial ligament insertion subperiostially with 4.5-mm notchplasty blade
9. Switch portals
10. Lateral visualization portal
11. Posterior instrumentation portal
12. Perform formal acromioplasty from posterior to anterior via sweeping medial to lateral movements using a 4.5-mm notchplasty blade
13. Acromioplasty complete when anterior acromial edge is posterior to anterior distal clavicle with smooth acromial undersurface
14. Remove inferior osteophytes from distal clavicle

the anterior portal, a 5.5-mm cannula is introduced over the arthroscopic cannula into the subacromial space. Inflow is positioned anteriorly and the scope is positioned posteriorly. The scope is withdrawn to a point just posterior to the anterior margin of the acromion. The inflow cannula is then pulled back to allow visualization within the subacromial space. If positioned appropriately, the arthroscope should now be within the "room with a view." Arthroscopic findings within the subacromial space that are consistent with chronic impingement lesions include hypertrophied and inflamed bursa, acromial undersurface abrasions, acromial and acromioclavicular osteophytes, hypertrophied coracoacromial ligament, and bursal side rotator cuff abrasions and tears (Fig. 15).

A lateral portal is then established approximately 3 cm lateral to the anterior edge of the acromion. The orientation of this portal is marked with an 18-gauge spinal needle visualized arthro-

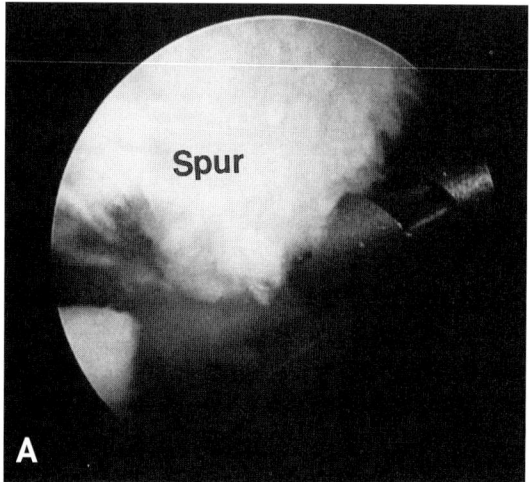
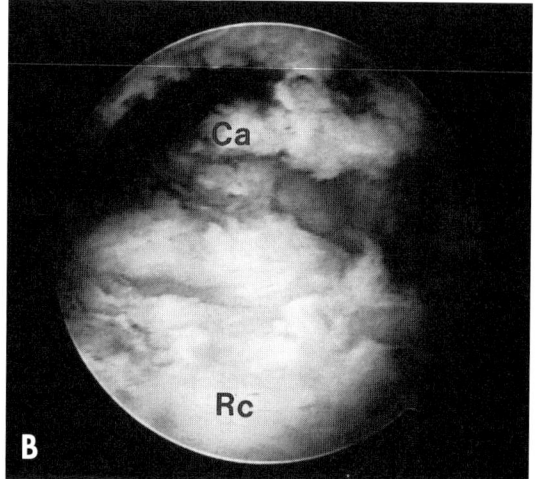

FIGURE 15
A, Arthroscopic view of prominent anterior acromial spur visualized from within the subacromial space. **B,** Arthroscopic view of bursal side partial-thickness rotator cuff tear prior to debridement.

scopically within the subacromial space to be perpendicular to the arthroscope and parallel to the underneath surface of the acromion. A 5.0-mm disposable cannula is then inserted into the subacromial space through this lateral portal for subacromial space instrumentation. Initially a subtotal bursectomy is done, using a 4.5 synovial resector, sweeping posteriorly to remove the posterior veil of synovial tissue, which is almost always present. During this portion of the procedure, the surgeon should be careful to avoid the medial and anterior aspect of the subacromial space to avoid bleeding, which typically is encountered when the soft tissues underlying the acromioclavicular (AC) joint are disturbed.

At this point, the bursal surface of the rotator cuff can be adequately inspected and any partial thickness bursal side tears can be debrided with the 4.5 synovial resector. A "kissing lesion"—matching fraying on the underside of the acromion and the superior side of the cuff—should be present (Fig. 16). If a full-thickness tear is encountered, its free edges are debrided with the synovial resector blade. Adhesions on the superior and inferior surfaces of the rotator cuff are released arthroscopically.

After completing debridement as needed, a 4.5-mm notchplasty burr is introduced through

the lateral portal and used to release the coracoacromial ligament from its bony insertion at the anterior edge of the acromion. The burr is first used to define the lateral edge of the acromion by gentle sweeping anterior to posterior movements to preserve the deltoid origin. Once the anterolateral corner of the acromion is defined, the burr is used to release the insertion of the coracoacromial ligament by successive gentle rolling move-

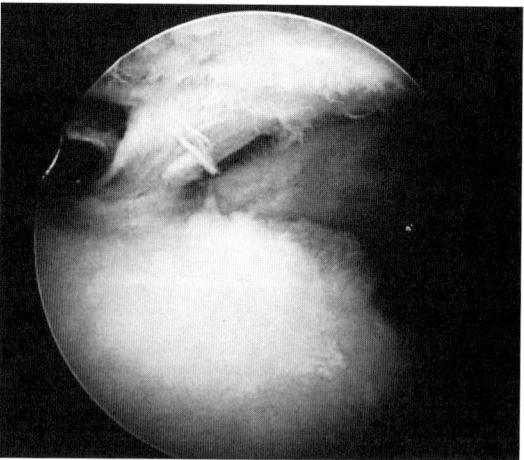

FIGURE 16
A "kissing lesion"—matched abrasion on the undersurface of the acromion and the superior/bursal surface of the rotator cuff—visualized from within the subacromial space.

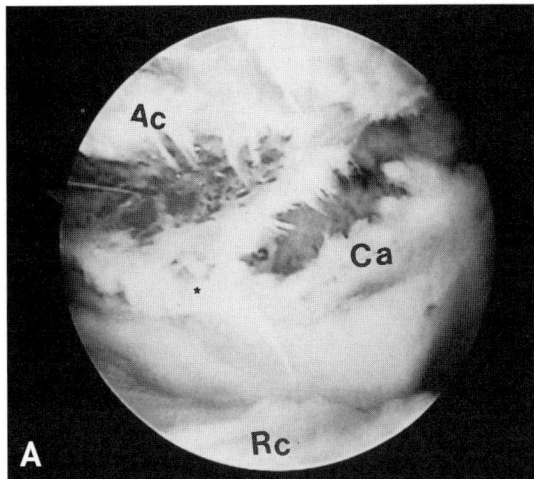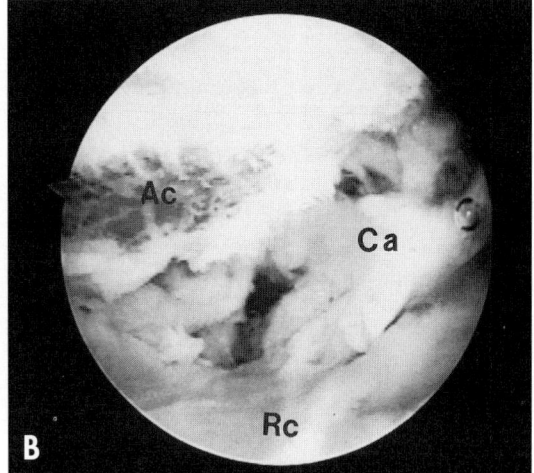

FIGURE 17
A, Partial detachment of coracoacromial (CA) ligament with 4.5-mm notchplasty blade. Note the intact slip of CA ligament to the acromioclavicular (AC) joint. **B,** Completed release of CA ligament. Note that the ligament drops inferiorly after release of slip to AC joint.

ments of the burr across the anterior edge of the acromion, from lateral to medial. Once the burr has reached the AC joint, a slip of the coracoacromial ligament can usually be seen inserting at the level of the AC joint (Fig. 17). Release of this slip by the described rolling motion allows the coracoacromial ligament to fall inferiorly from the anterior margin of the acromion.

If a full-thickness rotator cuff tear has been encountered, the burr is also used to debride the previous rotator cuff insertion site just lateral to the articular margin of the humeral head. Abrasion is limited to a depth of approximately 1 to 2 mm to allow for a strong bony bed where suture anchors are selected for repair.

Using "switching sticks," the posterior and lateral portals are switched. The arthroscope is inserted from the lateral portal and, while visualizing the anterior margin of the acromion, the notchplasty burr is inserted from the posterior portal and used to perform the formal acromioplasty. This technique permits contact of the instrument sheath with the posterior margin of the acromion, allowing for a smooth acromial resection and a flattened contour to the acromion in line with its posterior margin (Fig. 18). Bone is

resected by a series of sweeping movements of the burr from the medial to the lateral side, progressing from posterior to anterior. These movements are repeated until adequate acromial resection has been achieved. The surgeon must be

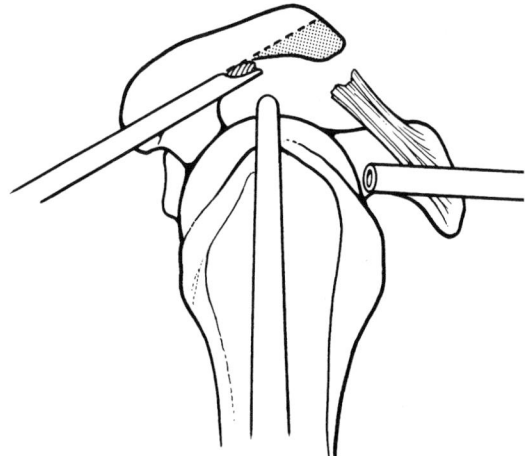

FIGURE 18
Line of resection for arthroscopic acromioplasty. Note portion of acromial undersurface to be resected from posterior to anterior using the posterior aspect of the acromion as a resection guide. Care must be taken to avoid amputation of bone anteriorly.

careful with the initial passages of the burr not to begin acromial resection too far posteriorly because this action may undermine anterior acromial osteophytes, resulting in loose bony fragments within the subacromial space. Adequate decompression has been achieved when the anterior aspect of the resected acromion is immediately posterior to the anterior aspect of the distal clavicle and the acromial undersurface lies on a flat plane with the posterior aspect of the acromion (Fig. 19). From this configuration, the inferior aspect of the distal clavicle and the AC joint can also be debrided if AC osteophytes are present. A cautery or other hemostatic device can be used to control bleeding during the procedure as necessary.

If a distal clavicle resection is to be performed, the anterior portal is repositioned for instrumentation of this area. Inflow is established posteriorly and a working portal is established through the previous anterior portal, just underneath the AC joint.

All instrumentation is then removed and excessive fluid is drained from the subacromial space. All portal sites are closed with steri-strips,

followed by injection of 0.25% bupivicaine with epinephrine into the portal sites, as well as into the subacromial space. Sterile bandages are applied to complete the procedure.

ARTHROSCOPIC DISTAL CLAVICLE RESECTION

Arthroscopic distal clavicle resection can be performed either directly or indirectly. Direct resection involves introducing the arthroscope and arthroscopic instruments into the anterior and posterior aspects of the AC joint without violating the underlying subacromial space. Proponents of this approach feel it is preferable in isolated AC disease because there is no added surgical trauma to the subacromial space and excellent visualization of the distal clavicle is afforded.[42,51,56] Disadvantages include the inability to use these portals for anything other than distal clavicle resection. Also, a 2.7-mm arthroscope and smaller burrs and shavers must be used initially in most cases before progressing to a standard arthroscope and working instruments.[57]

Indirect arthroscopic distal clavicle resection is performed with the arthroscope and working instruments positioned within the subacromial

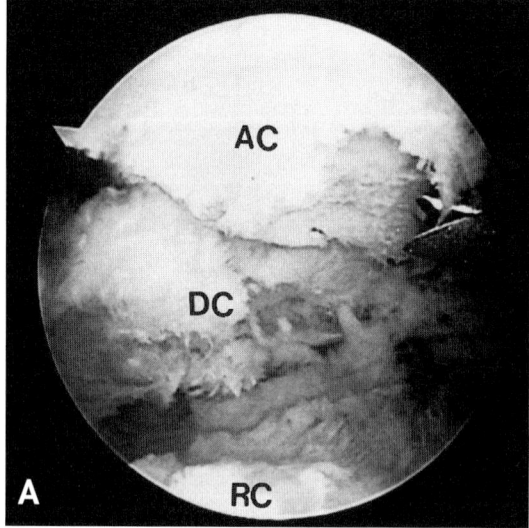
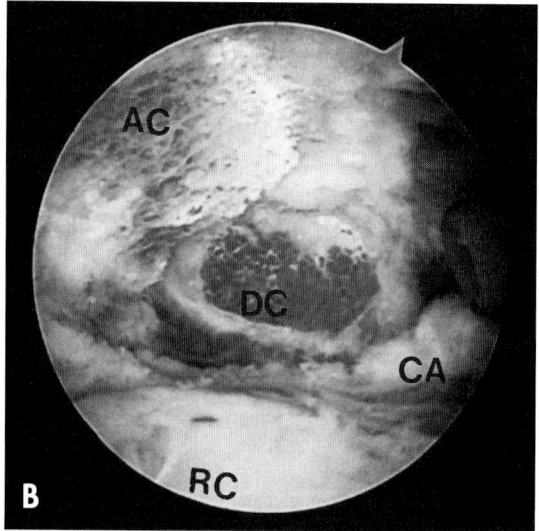

FIGURE 19
A, Partially completed acromioplasty. Arthroscope is positioned in the lateral portal and notchplasty blade in the posterior portal. Acromioplasty is proceeding from posterior to anterior in this left shoulder. **B,** Completed acromioplasty as visualized from the lateral portal. Note that the anterior margin of the resected acromion is posterior to the anterior margin of the distal clavicle in this right shoulder.

space, through previously established portals. Because distal clavicle resection usually is performed in conjunction with other surgical procedures (ie, arthroscopic subacromial decompression), no additional surgical trauma is induced. Proponents of the indirect technique cite the importance of arthroscopic glenohumeral and subacromial inspection, given the high incidence of associated pathology.[15]

Johnson[84] initially reported the direct superior approach to the distal clavicle in 1986. In 1992, Flatow and associates[42] gave a detailed account of this technique. The patient is placed in a beach chair position and 22-gauge needles are used to determine the location and orientation of the AC joint before beginning the procedure. This step is extremely important when using this technique, because the inclination of the AC joint varies among individuals. The AC joint is then distended with normal saline solution.

An anterior superior portal and a posterior superior portal are used; each is located approximately 0.75 cm from the joint and positioned in line with the AC joint (Fig. 20). Initially, the 2.7-mm wrist arthroscope is positioned through the posterior superior portal. The anterior superior portal is used as a working portal. A 2-mm resector is passed through this portal and used to

debride the AC joint, exposing the bony edges of the medial acromion and the distal clavicle. A 2-mm burr is then used to widen the joint space to allow use of the standard 4-mm arthroscope and larger resection instruments.

Using electrocautery, the periosteum is elevated from the circumference of the distal clavicle in order to preserve the capsule and ligamentous structures. This step provides full exposure of the distal clavicle, allowing an even resection. The resection is completed with larger burrs and arthroscopic rasps. The arthroscope is switched to the anterior portal to assure complete bony resection. A probe may also be used to confirm the absence of overhanging ridges of bone. Upon completion of the procedure, the joint is injected with long-acting anesthetic agent and the portals are closed with subcuticular suture.

Early descriptions of this technique involve the removal of 1 to 1.5 cm of bone from the distal clavicle.[42] Subsequent studies report equally satisfactory results obtained with resection of as little as 5 to 7 mm of bone, as long as the AC joint is stable and the resection is even.[51,56] This technique does not surgically violate the glenohumeral or subacromial space although the spaces are diagnostically evaluated. This factor is felt to be an advantage by Flatow and associates[42] and is their

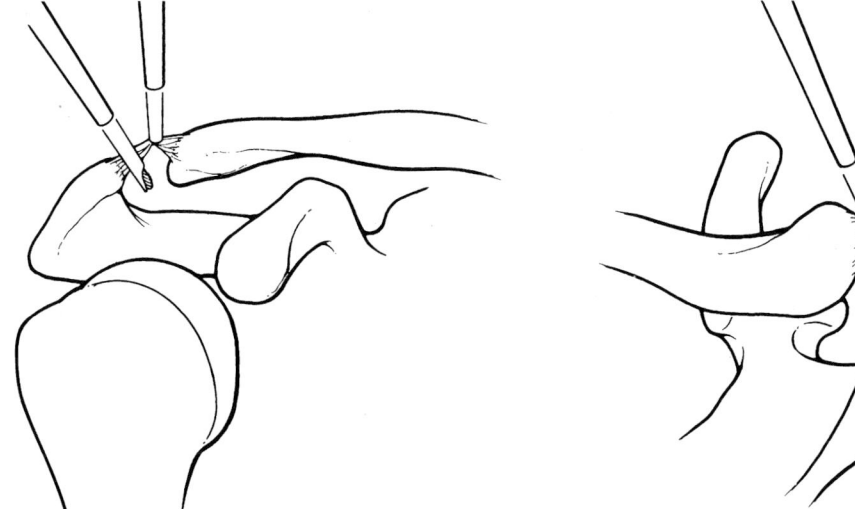

FIGURE 20
Portal configuration for direct superior approach to distal clavicle resection. Anterior view **(left)** and superior view **(right).**

preferred technique, only in isolated AC disease. They and others prefer a subacromial approach when subacromial decompression is required.

The indirect approach to distal clavicle resection was initially proposed by Ellman[20] in 1987 and Esch and associates[55] in 1988. Various authors using this technique have documented successful results.[41,50,57,58,85] The indirect approach to distal clavicle excision is our favored approach (Outline 2). The majority of our distal clavicle resections follow arthroscopic subacromial decompression. Anesthesia, patient positioning techniques, and position of the shoulder are unchanged from our standard arthroscopic acromioplasty technique. Upon completion of the acromioplasty, a standard arthroscope remains positioned in the lateral portal with inflow through a 5.0-mm cannula anteriorly. The posterior portal was used for instrumentation during the arthroscopic acromioplasty. A single switching stick is used to change inflow to the posterior portal.

Through the previously established anterior portal, a blunt 5.0-mm disposable cannula is introduced through the deltoid muscle soft spot directly in line with and underneath the AC joint (Fig. 21). Introduction of this cannula is visualized with the arthroscope. This anterior portal is then used as an instrumentation portal. Rotating the arthroscopic lens posteriorly, a direct "down the line" view of the AC joint can be obtained. A 4.5-mm notchplasty burr is then introduced through the anterior portal. The medial facet of the acromion is resected first to allow access to the entire articular surface of the distal clavicle.

This notchplasty burr is then used for formal distal clavicle resection. The superior portion of the distal clavicle is excised first, using a sweeping posterior to anterior technique. The underlying inferior distal clavicle can then be resected using a series of superior to inferior sweeping motions to maintain a smooth line of resection. The sequence can be repeated until distal clavicle resection is adequate (minimum 6 to 7 mm). Approximately 1 cm of the distal clavicle can be resected before the superior capsule tapers to a thin, less viable structure (Fig. 22). This "thinning

OUTLINE 2

STEPS OF INDIRECT ARTHROSCOPIC DISTAL CLAVICLE RESECTION

1. Maintain lateral decubitus position after arthroscopic acromioplasty
2. Maintain arthroscope through lateral portal
3. Switch inflow to posterior portal and use anterior portal for instrumentation
4. Resect medial facet of acromion with 4.5-mm notchplasty blade
5. Perform formal distal clavicle resection with 4.5-mm notchplasty blade, carefully maintaining superior capsule and ligaments
6. Confirm resection of approximately 1 cm of the distal clavicle

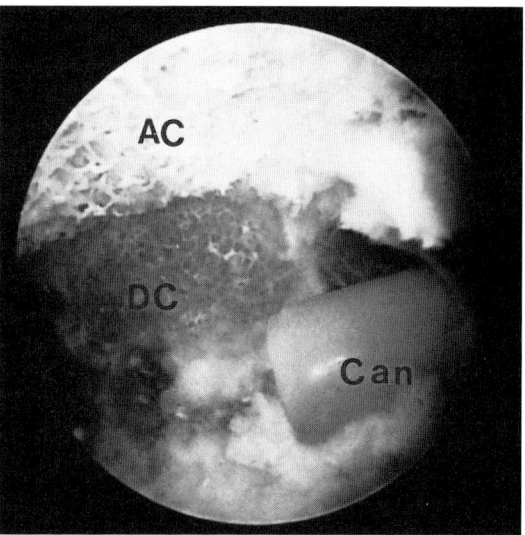

FIGURE 21
Cannula positioned in line with acromioclavicular joint through deltoid muscle soft spot via the anterior portal for indirect technique of distal clavicle resection. Arthroscope is positioned in the lateral portal in this right shoulder.

out" of the superior capsule can be visualized arthroscopically. Resection length can be checked using the known width of the 5.0-mm disposable cannula. At this point, a Holmium: YAG laser or electrocautery can be inserted from the anterior portal and used to seal the bony surfaces of the distal clavicle and the medial acromion. The laser

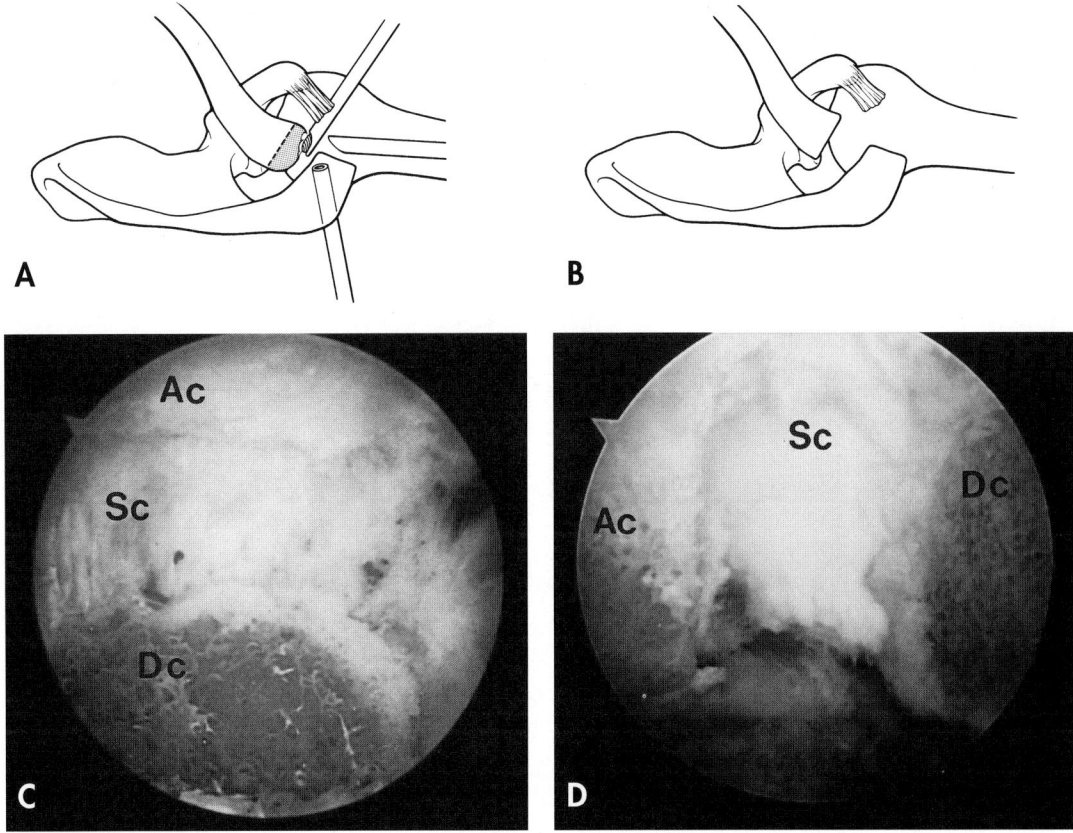

FIGURE 22

A, Portal configuration for indirect approach to distal clavicle resection. **B,** Completed acromioplasty and distal clavicle resection. **C,** "End on" view of distal clavicle resection with arthroscope positioned through the lateral portal. Note that the integrity of the superior acromioclavicular capsule is maintained. **D,** Anterior view of distal clavicle resection with arthroscope positioned through the anterior portal. Superior AC capsule remains intact.

can also be used to thicken and tension the superior and posterior capsular structures of the AC joint. We believe this should provide increased stability to the AC joint postoperatively. At this point, all instrumentation is removed. Arthroscopic portals are closed with steri-strips, completing the procedure.

ROTATOR CUFF REPAIR

Regardless of the method of rotator cuff repair, we believe arthroscopy is indicated first. This order allows for evaluation and treatment of concomitant glenohumeral lesions as well as the performance of arthroscopic acromioplasty and distal clavicle resection if indicated. Once the steps

involved in the arthroscopic acromioplasty and distal clavicle resection have been completed, we proceed with evaluation and treatment of the rotator cuff tear.

With the arthroscope positioned in the posterior portal and inflow established anteriorly, the lateral portal is used for instrumentation. The torn edge of the rotator cuff is debrided to viable tendinous edges. The size of the tear and quality of the remaining tendon are assessed. An arthroscopic grabber can be passed through the lateral portal and used to advance the rotator cuff tendon laterally to its insertion at the greater tuberosity (Fig. 23), thereby allowing assessment of both the quality of the tendon and its excursion.

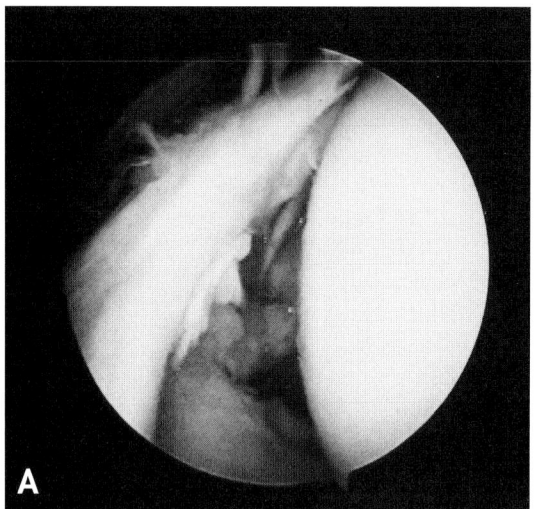 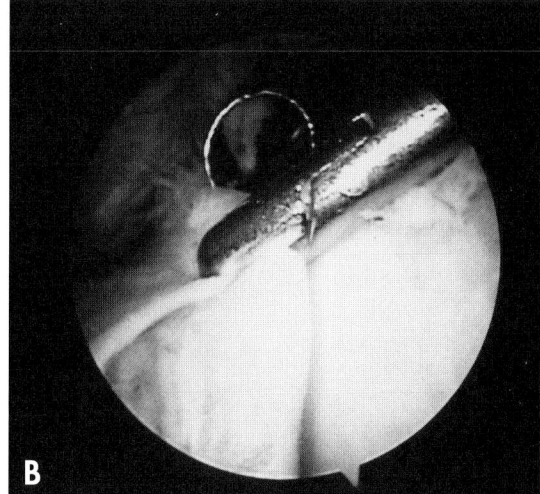

FIGURE 23
A, Large full-thickness rotator cuff tear "at rest" as visualized through the lateral portal. **B,** Determination of rotator cuff tendon quality and excursion using arthroscopic grabber positioned from the posterior portal to advance the tendon laterally to its insertion at the greater tuberosity.

Additional mobilization of the tendon can be achieved by releasing soft tissues from both the bursal and articular surfaces of the rotator cuff. The coracohumeral ligament can be carefully released with use of an arthroscopic resector passed through the lateral portal. A capsular release can also be performed under direct visualization with an elevator positioned through the lateral portal.

Proceeding by the indications mentioned earlier, the method of rotator cuff repair is then chosen. Regardless of which technique is used for repair, the position of the patient remains unchanged.

Arthroscopic Rotator Cuff Repair
If the rotator cuff tear is amenable to arthroscopic repair, an arthroscopic 4.5-mm notchplasty burr is introduced through the lateral portal and used to lightly abrade the greater tuberosity just lateral to the articular surface. This arthroscopic abrasion creates a bleeding surface, but resection to cancellous bone is avoided. Using an 18-gauge spinal needle passed just lateral to the anterior acromion, a direct path is created to this "trough." A small superolateral stab incision is made to allow access of instruments. A variety of suture anchors have been proposed for repair of the rotator cuff. Regardless of the anchor system, repair is performed by either a transtendon technique or an "anchor first" technique.

In the transtendon technique, the suture anchor is placed in a "blind" fashion. With the arthroscope in the posterior portal, the appropriate sites for suture anchors are identified anteriorly and posteriorly. Depending on the anchor system used, a drill or an awl is introduced through the superolateral portal under direct visualization. A pilot hole is then created at the appropriate anchor site (Fig. 24, *A*). The anchor is then introduced through the superolateral portal to confirm appropriate alignment with the pilot hole (Fig. 24, *B*). An arthroscopic grabber is inserted through the lateral portal and used to advance the rotator cuff tendon laterally over the previously drilled pilot hole. The suture anchor is then inserted through the rotator cuff tendon into the hole. Upon final seating of the anchor, the introduction device is removed and both suture arms are positioned through the rotator cuff and out the superolateral portal (Fig. 24, *C*). These are secured with a hemostat and this procedure is repeated for other suture

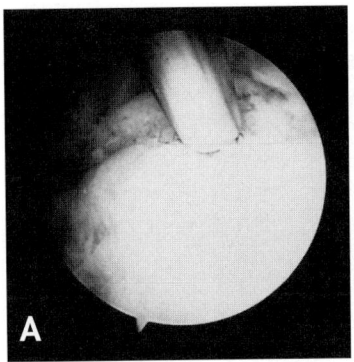 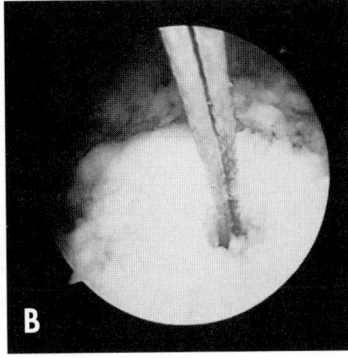 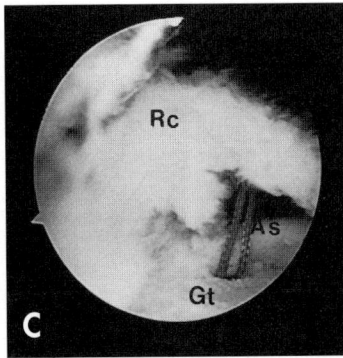

FIGURE 24
A, An awl is positioned through the superolateral portal to create a pilot hole within the abraded greater tuberosity (Gt) for subsequent anchor placement. **B,** Anchor passed through the superolateral portal to confirm appropriate ligament with the pilot hole. **C,** Anchor fully seated within the pilot hole after transtendinous placement through the rotator cuff tendon. Note both arms of the suture are through the rotator cuff tendon

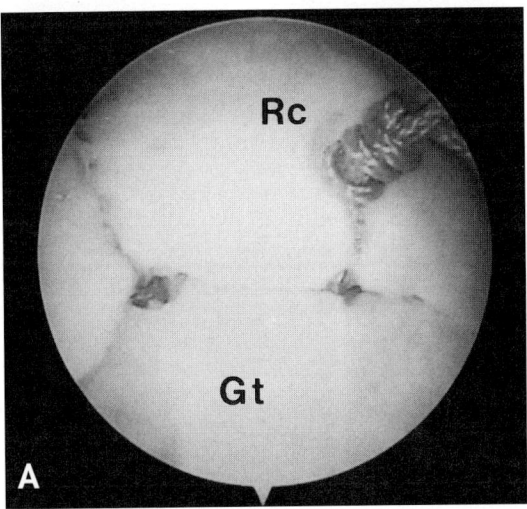 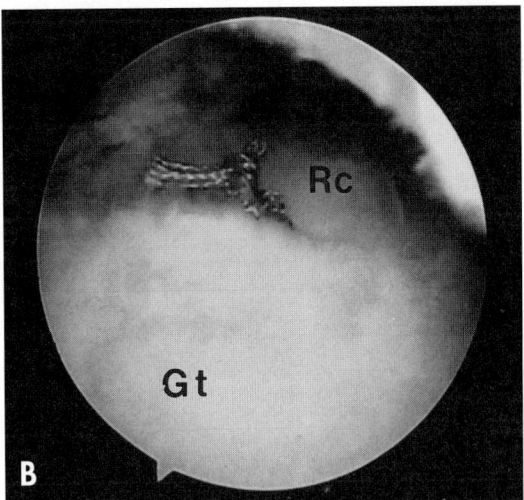

FIGURE 25
A, Arthroscopic rotator cuff repair using simple suture technique. Arthroscope is positioned within the lateral portal.
B, Arthroscopic rotator cuff repair using mattress suture technique. Arthroscope is positioned within the lateral portal.

anchor sites. Typically, two anchors are adequate for tears that are appropriate for arthroscopic fixation. Sutures can then be tied in either a simple or mattress fashion using arthroscopic knot tying techniques.

If simple sutures are chosen, a crochet hook is inserted through the lateral portal and used to retrieve a single arm of each suture from the articular side of the rotator cuff, leaving only a single arm of each suture passing through the cuff ten-

don. Paired sutures can then be retrieved through either the lateral portal or the superolateral portal and tied arthroscopically, achieving simple suture repair of the rotator cuff (Fig. 25, *A*).

If mattress sutures are chosen, a crochet hook is introduced from the lateral portal and used to retrieve a single arm of each suture from the superior (bursal) surface of the rotator cuff. These individual suture arms from separate suture anchors are then tied externally through the lateral portal and advanced back into the subacromial space by firmly pulling the superior suture limbs. This procedure provides a single mattress suture. The superior suture arms are then retrieved through the lateral portal and tied using arthroscopic knot tying techniques for completion of a double mattress suture (Fig. 25, *B*).

When performing the "anchor first" technique, the configuration of arthroscopic instruments remains the same. The pilot hole is initiated as previously described (Fig. 26, *A*). In this technique, however, the rotator cuff tendon is not advanced laterally before anchor placement, allowing direct visualization of the pilot hole for insertion of the suture anchor (Fig. 26, *B*). After anchor insertion, suture arms must then be retrieved through the rotator cuff tendon. If a simple suture technique is used, only a single suture arm need be retrieved through the edge of the rotator cuff tendon. If a mattress suture is to be placed, then both suture arms should be retrieved through the rotator cuff tendon at appropriately spaced intervals (Fig. 27). These sutures can be retrieved using either a suture retriever passed

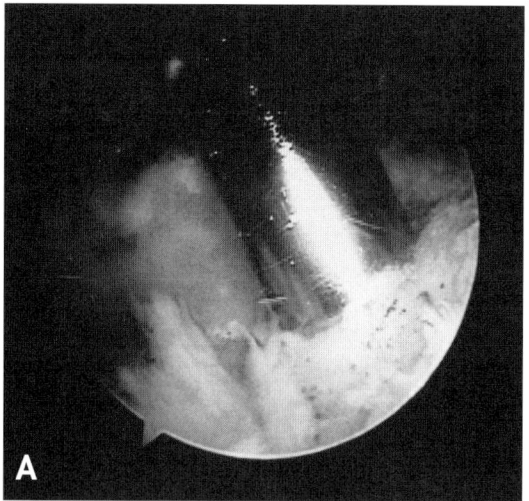 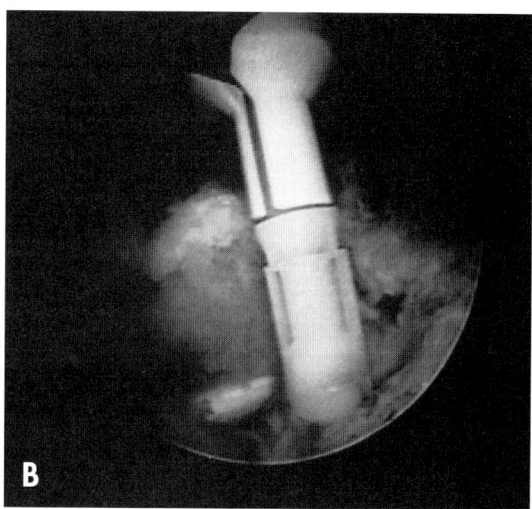

FIGURE 26
A, A drill hole is created in the abraded greater tuberosity for subsequent suture anchor placement. **B,** Anchor is placed directly into the pilot hole (not transtendinous) when using the "anchor first" technique.

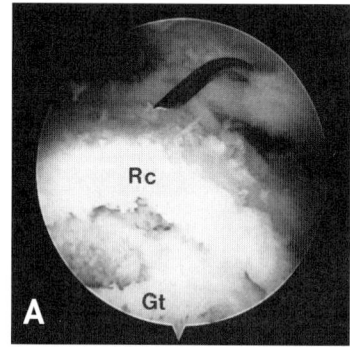 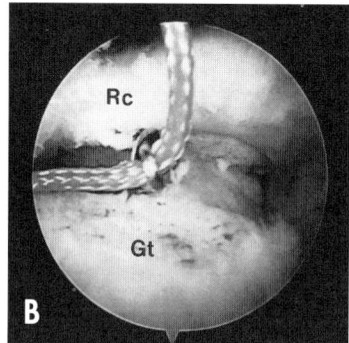 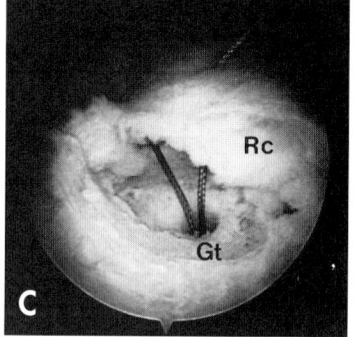

FIGURE 27
Technique of suture retrieval after suture anchor is placed directly into bone. **A,** Suture retriever about to pierce through rotator cuff tendon from superior to inferior surface. **B,** Retriever through the rotator cuff tendon, grabbing a single arm of the previously placed suture. **C,** Suture arms retrieved through tendon in a horizontal mattress fashion.

through the appropriate portal, or by the suture shuttle technique using a suture punch (Linvatec, Largo, FL). Once these suture arms are retrieved through the tendon, they are tied using arthroscopic knot tying techniques to achieve secure rotator cuff repair.

Stollsteimer and Savoie[76] note that assessment of the repair is an ongoing process. The three most important evaluation points include ensuring adequate excursion and quality of the tendon, adequate suture anchor purchase within the bone, and direct visual inspection of the rotator cuff upon final repair. After placement of each suture anchor, purchase should be tested by applying gentle traction to the suture arms to ensure adequate stability at the bone-anchor interface. Upon completion of repair, the repair site should be inspected with the arthroscope from both the posterior and the lateral portals. Adequate apposition of tendon to bone should be confirmed by direct visualization and by probing techniques. If the repair is judged inadequate, sutures and suture anchors must be removed and repair must be reinitiated using either arthroscopic techniques or progressing to a mini-open repair.

Mini-Open Rotator Cuff Repair

If the dimensions and characteristics of the rotator cuff tear are such that arthroscopic repair is not feasible, then progression to a mini-open rotator cuff repair may be necessary. These tears should, however, still fall within the above mentioned parameters. The patient is maintained in the lateral decubitus position, and traction is continually applied to the upper extremity. The standard technique of mini-open rotator cuff repair was detailed by Levy and associates[66] in 1990, and by Paulos and Kody[75] in 1994, with subsequent modifications by Liu and Baker.[72–74] Our technique is a modification of those previously described.

After arthroscopic subacromial decompression and distal clavicle resection have been performed as indicated, the area of incision is located off the anterolateral border of the resected acromion with an 18-gauge spinal needle placed percutaneously (Fig. 28, *A*). After the tear has been localized, a 2- to 3-cm incision is begun at the anterolateral border of the acromion and extended distally. Rarely do we need to extend this incision into the previously established lateral portal (Fig. 28, *B*). This incision is carried sharply to the deltoid fascia, which is then incised longitudinally. The origin of the deltoid remains intact. The fibers of the deltoid are split longitudinally using blunt dissection. Spreading begins at the anterolateral corner of the acromion and extends distally for not more than 4 cm to preserve the integrity of the axillary nerve. A self-retaining retractor can then

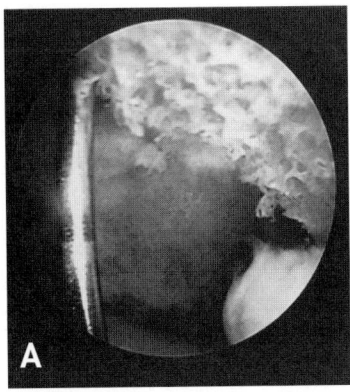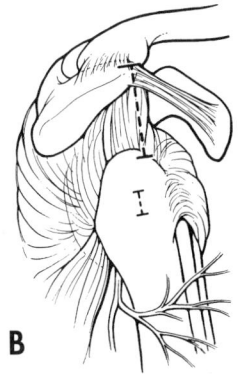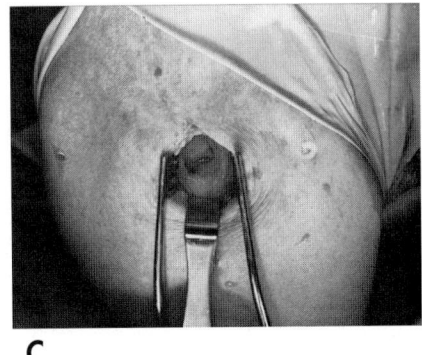

FIGURE 28

A, Localization of incision for mini-open rotator cuff repair using an 18-gauge spinal needle percutaneously placed at the anterolateral border of the resected acromion. **B,** Line of incision. This incision should not be extended beyond 4 cm from the lateral edge of the acromion to avoid risk of axillary nerve injury. **C,** Photograph of mini-open approach to rotator cuff repair. Rotator cuff tear is exposed within the wound. Note that incision does not extend as far laterally as the lateral portal.

be inserted within this split in the deltoid to allow visualization of the rotator cuff tear (Fig. 28, *C*). Any remaining hypertrophied bursal tissue or devitalized tendon edges can now be removed.

The rotator cuff tendons can then be repaired in either a tendon to tendon or a tendon to bone fashion. Defects within the rotator cuff that are primarily longitudinal in orientation can be repaired in a tendon to tendon fashion using a running nonabsorbable suture. Paulos and Kody[75] take this suture through paired transosseous tunnels laterally for added security.

The majority of rotator cuff tears require tendon to bone repair. Once exposure has been obtained, a rongeur may be used to decorticate the greater tuberosity just lateral to the articular surface if this was not done arthroscopically. Once a cancellous trough has been prepared, either transosseous tunnels or suture anchors may be used for tendon repair.

Recent studies show suture anchors to be equivalent or superior to transosseous tunnel fixation.[86,87] Hecker and associates[86] demonstrated that the primary mode of failure was by the suture tearing out through the tendon rather than failure of the anchor itself. Using fresh frozen cadavers, Reed and associates[87] evaluated the pullout strength of repair through transosseous tunnels as compared to suture anchors. They found the strength of the suture anchors to be significantly greater than that of the transosseous tunnels. They also demonstrated that the primary mode of failure was by suture breakage. It was concluded that suture anchors provided superior fixation of the rotator cuff.

The positioning of these anchors is very important in determining pullout strength. They should be directed into the subchondral bone adjacent to the articular surface, and they should be countersunk so there is no excessive irritation to the undersurface of the rotator cuff. In 1995, Burkhart[88] described the "deadman theory," which biomechanically rationalizes the optimal placement of suture anchors in order to increase their pullout strength and reduce suture tension. Basically, the anchors are placed such that the line of pull of the rotator cuff is approximately

90° to the alignment of the anchor with the humerus abducted 30°. The stability of these anchors is greatly influenced by the quality of bone in which they are placed. Placement of each anchor should be tested to confirm adequate fixation at the bone-anchor interface.

Typically, #2 or larger braided nonabsorbable sutures are used for repair. Although Burkhart (personal communication, Atlanta, GA, 1996) found that two simple sutures were stronger than a single mattress suture, Gerber and associates[89] noted simple sutures to be significantly less effective than mattress sutures. They, therefore, recommended that simple sutures be used only for small tears that are not under significant tension.

The decision to use transosseous tunnels or suture anchors is ultimately based on surgeon preference. Tunnels or anchors are positioned so that the tendon edges will be advanced to the bony trough. We use sutures placed in a modified Southern California Orthopaedic Institute (SCOI) or a modified Mason-Allen technique in order to attain a more secure grasp of the tendon edge[90] (Fig. 29). The sutures typically are advanced through transosseous tunnels (Fig. 30) and tied over the lateral edge of the greater tuberosity so they do not protrude into the subacromial space (Fig. 31). This completes rotator cuff repair. The deltoid fascia is closed with a running absorbable suture. Subcutaneous and skin closure complete the procedure.

Open Rotator Cuff Repair

Tears that are too large or have inadequate tissues to be repaired by arthroscopic or mini-open techniques require formal open rotator cuff repair. The patient remains in the lateral decubitus position and traction is continually applied to the involved upper extremity, providing increased working space within the acromiohumeral interval. Arthroscopic inspection of the rotator cuff tear should confirm that an open repair is indicated. Under direct arthroscopic visualization, the anterolateral corner of the acromion is marked with an 18-gauge spinal needle. This marks the site of skin incision. Arthroscopic instrumentation is then removed from the subacromial space.

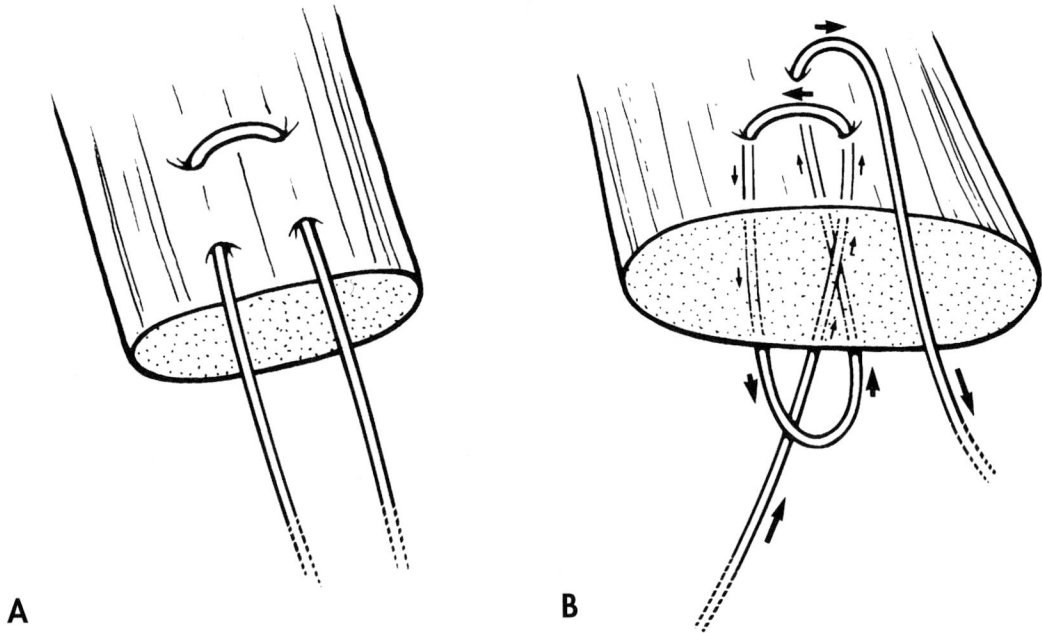

A   **B**

FIGURE 29
A, Illustration of the modified Southern California Orthopaedic Institute (SCOI) technique of suture placement.
B, Illustration of the modified Mason-Allen technique of suture placement.

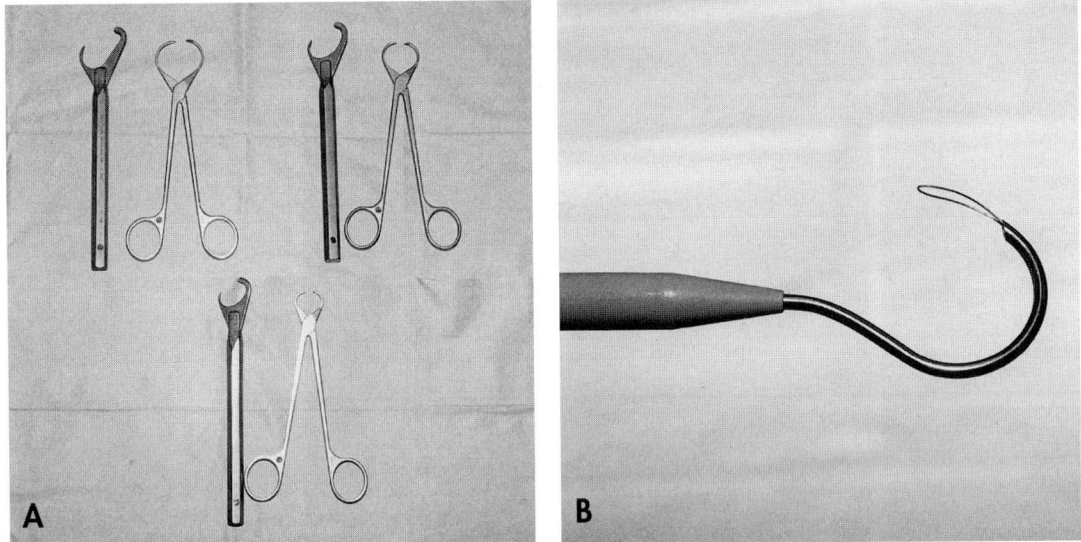

A   **B**

FIGURE 30
The concept rotator cuff repair system used for creation of transosseous tunnels (Linvatec, Largo, FL). **A,** Cortical gauges and circular rasps in three different sizes. **B,** Circular suture retriever also available in three different sizes.

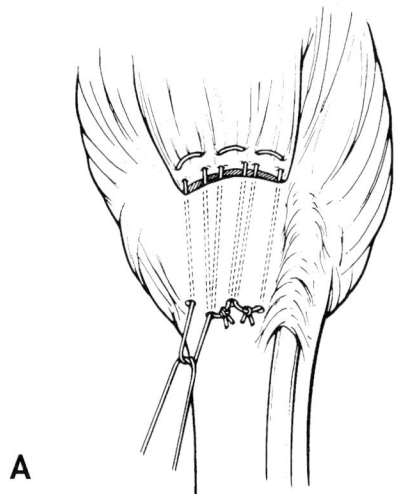
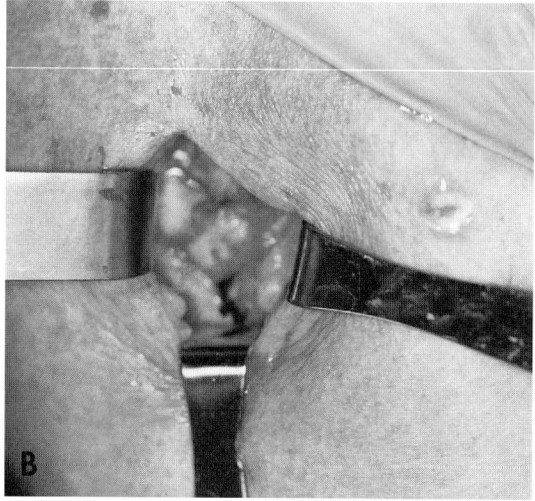

FIGURE 31
A, Completion of repair of a large rotator cuff tear using transosseous tunnels and sutures placed in a modified Southern California Orthopaedic Institute technique. **B,** Photograph of completed rotator cuff repair using transosseous tunnels.

An incision is begun at the acromioclavicular (AC) joint and extended along the anterior border of the acromion, proceeding laterally for a distance of approximately 5 cm. This incision is taken sharply through the skin and subcutaneous tissues. The deltoid origin is then taken down from the anterior border of the acromion. A self-retaining retractor is then inserted, providing excellent exposure of the rotator cuff tear. Remaining hypertrophied bursal tissues and devitalized tendons are removed.

Mobilization of the rotator cuff tear is completed by releasing any soft-tissue attachments on the bursal or articular surface of the rotator cuff tendons. Once adequate mobilization of the cuff tendons has been achieved, a bony trough is fashioned just lateral to the articular surface of the humeral head in the area of the tendon defect. The configuration of the cuff tear is evaluated for subsequent placement of sutures. Again, for these larger tears we use a modified SCOI or a modified Mason-Allen technique of suture placement.[91] The most anterior of these sutures is typically used to close the rotator interval.

Once again, the decision to use anchors or transosseous tunnels is one of surgeon prefer-ence. Abrams and Burkhead (personal communication, Amelia Island, FL, 1996) have advocated the use of transosseous tunnels centrally with anchors placed at the anterior and posterior edges of the tear for augmentation of fixation. This is an effort to biomechanically reproduce the cable crescent formation described by Burkhart.[91] Whether using anchors or transosseous tunnels, the tendon edges should be advanced into the bony trough to complete repair.

In individuals in whom large rotator cuff tears are repaired, the coracoacromial ligament is repaired. This ligament is repaired with #2 braided nonabsorbable suture to soft tissues at the medial aspect of the acromion in order to help prevent humeral head migration should the repair not heal or the cuff not function to keep the humeral head centered in the glenoid fossa.

Attention is then directed toward repair of the deltoid origin. Although various methods exist, we use a technique of advancement of the origin superiorly, recreating the normal rounded contour of the anterior shoulder. Braided nonabsorbable sutures are used in a pants-over-vest fashion, securing the deltoid origin to the delto-trapezial fascia overlying the acromion and

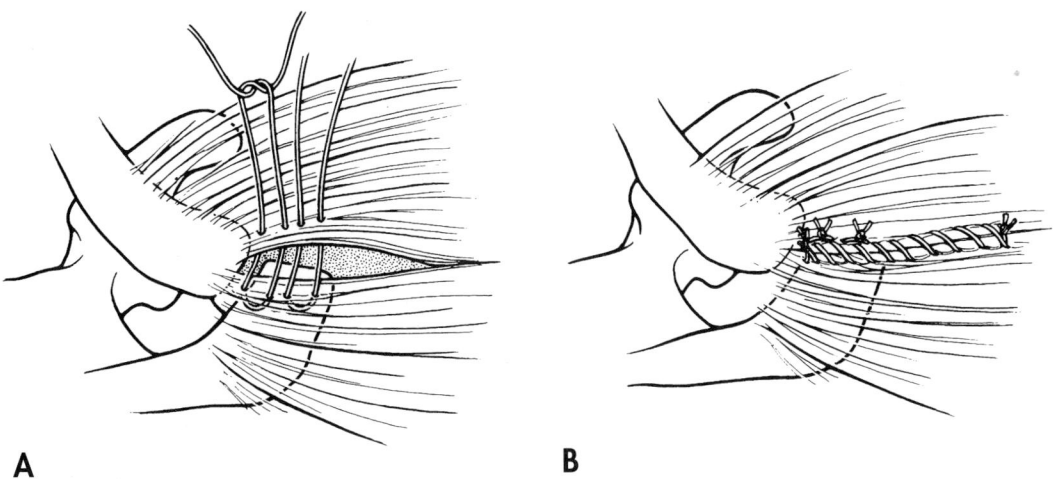

A   **B**

FIGURE 32
A, Deltoid origin repair is anchored to deltotrapezial fascia using pants-over-vest technique with braided #2 nonabsorbable suture. **B,** Completion of deltoid repair. In addition to pants-over-vest sutures, repair is reinforced with running #1 absorbable monofilament suture.

AC joint. This suture line is then reinforced with #1 absorbable polydioxanone suture. The longitudinal incision in the deltoid fascia is closed similarly, completing the deltoid repair (Fig. 32). Subcutaneous and skin closure is then performed.

POSTOPERATIVE CARE

ACROMIOPLASTY AND ACROMIOCLAVICULAR RESECTION

Rehabilitation can proceed more rapidly after arthroscopic acromioplasty than after open acromioplasty. Hand, wrist, and elbow exercises are begun on the day of surgery. Patients are initially placed in a sling for comfort with active range of motion exercises begun as early as tolerated. The sling is usually discarded within the first 3 to 4 days. Resistance exercises in abduction are delayed for 2 to 3 weeks, but rotation and flexion are initiated immediately. Patients typically progress to activities of daily living within the first 2 to 3 weeks, with return to sports activities or manual labor delayed for 2 to 3 months. Adding arthroscopic distal clavicle resection to the acromioplasty procedure influences postoper-

ative rehabilitation very little, and the same general protocol is followed.

ROTATOR CUFF REPAIR

Rehabilitation after rotator cuff repair proceeds similarly whether or not deltoid detachment is required. With the deltoid securely repaired, no modification is needed. Although we may be somewhat more liberal after repair of small rotator cuff tears, our general rehabilitation scheme is as follows. Initially the patient is placed in an abduction pillow to improve blood supply to the critical zone of the rotator cuff and to protect and relax the repair for a period of up to 1 week. At 1 week, passive forward flexion is begun and the patient is placed in an abduction sling for daytime activities with maintenance of the pillow at night. Over the next 2 to 3 weeks, active assisted motion is begun, including external rotation and forward flexion. Full passive mobilization is initiated by the fourth week with progression to active rotator cuff exercises. Strengthening of the rotator cuff against resistance begins at about 6 to 8 weeks with progression to functional activities typically by 3 months postoperatively.

COMPLICATIONS

Several isolated complications of shoulder arthroscopy have been reported, although the incidence of these in any one series has remained very low. More important complications noted in the past have included uncontrolled bleeding,[24] deltoid damage with over aggressive anterior and anterolateral acromial resection,[27,40] contralateral lateral femoral cutaneous nerve palsy,[24] axillary nerve palsy,[15] postoperative acromion fracture,[15] superficial infection,[23] and adhesive capsulitis.[92] Other less significant complications have included transient dysesthesias, localized hematomas, loosening or breakage of equipment, standard anesthetic postoperative complications, and fluid extravasation. We feel that with attention to detail most of these complications can be avoided.

RESULTS

ARTHROSCOPIC ACROMIOPLASTY

Results of arthroscopic subacromial decompression are similar to those of open acromioplasty. When performing arthroscopic acromioplasty for advanced stage II impingement or for partial thickness rotator cuff tears, satisfactory results range from 76% to 100%[14,20,24,27,55,83,92] (Table 1).

In 1987 Ellman[20] reported the results of his initial 50 patients. Forty of these had a diagnosis of stage II impingement and ten had stage III (rotator cuff tear) disease. Using the UCLA shoulder rating scale, 88% satisfactory results were obtained with only 12% unsatisfactory results. In a second report in 1991,[23] he reported the 2- to 5-year follow-up of 65 patients treated by arthroscopic acromioplasty. All patients in this group

TABLE 1

PERCENTAGE OF SATISFACTORY RESULTS AFTER ARTHROSCOPIC ACROMIOPLASTY

Reference	Follow-up	Stage II Disease	Partial Thickness Tear	Full Thickness Tear
20	1 to 3 years	90%*		80%
55	19 months	82%	76%	77%
24	29 to 31 months	91%	82.5%	56%
14	17 months	83%	66%	60%
23	2 to 5 years	89%*		
34	1 year minimum	90%*		
26	20.3 months	88%*		
63	24.6 months			84%
22	32.2 months	83%		
27	23 months	86%	86%	55%
30	12 months	> 90%		
93	27.7 months	81%	81%	77%
79	45.8 months			68%
25	41 months	94%	95%†	

* Includes partial thickness tears
† Includes full thickness tears < 1 cm

had stage II disease. Using the same rating system, 89% satisfactory results were achieved. Ellman and Kay[23] concluded that arthroscopic acromioplasty was an acceptable alternative to open subacromial decompression.

In 1990, Paulos and Franklin[15] reviewed 80 consecutive arthroscopic subacromial decompressions in 76 patients with an average follow-up of 32 months. Diagnoses included stage II impingement in 42 shoulders and stage III impingement in 38 shoulders. Final results showed 85% of patients satisfied with their procedure, with over 80% of patients returning to sports activities at their preinjury level of competition. This report also documented the high incidence of unsuspected associated pathologic lesions; 59 patients in this series were found to have an additional lesion. The authors concluded arthroscopic acromioplasty to be highly effective in the treatment of impingement syndrome without a full-thickness rotator cuff tear, but recommended open repair of full-thickness tears in active patients.

In 1990, Gartsman[24] reported his results with arthroscopic subacromial decompression in 154 shoulders. Of these, 89 had stage II impingement syndrome, 40 had partial-thickness rotator cuff tears, and 25 had full-thickness rotator cuff tears. Unsatisfactory results were documented in 11 of the 25 patients with full-thickness rotator cuff tears. Among the 40 patients with partial-thickness tears, seven unsatisfactory results were obtained. Two of these resulted from a technically inadequate procedure; the other five were attributed to worker's compensation. Among the 89 patients with stage II impingement, 11 unsatisfactory results were obtained. Eight of these resulted from a technically inadequate procedure. Gartsman[24] concluded arthroscopic acromioplasty was an effective technique for isolated stage II impingement syndrome and for partial-thickness rotator cuff tears.

Altchek and associates[14] reported results of 40 patients with a minimum follow-up of 12 months. Twenty-four of these patients had stage II impingement, six had partial-thickness cuff tears, and ten had full-thickness cuff tears. Satisfactory results were obtained in 73% of the entire patient population. This included 20 of 24 patients with stage II impingement, four of six with partial-thickness tears, and six of ten with full-thickness tears. The average time to return to work was 9 days, with full recovery averaging 3.8 months.

In 1992, Burns and Turba[22] reported results of arthroscopic subacromial decompression in 29 patients over a 32-month follow-up period. Results were evaluated using the UCLA shoulder rating scale, with 82% of patients having a satisfactory result. Of the college athletes in this series, only 56% were able to return to their preoperative activity levels, at an average of 6.6 months postoperatively. A high incidence of associated pathology was again noted in this series, with 79% of patients undergoing treatment for an additional abnormality.

In comparisons of open versus arthroscopic acromioplasty, superior results of the arthroscopic technique have been demonstrated. In 1989, Norlin[29] reported a prospective comparison of ten patients decompressed by arthroscopic technique and ten patients decompressed by open technique. At 3 months' follow-up, the arthroscopic group showed more rapid rehabilitation and better range of motion than did the open group.

In 1992, Van Holsbeeck and associates[28] detailed a retrospective study of 53 patients undergoing open decompression versus 53 patients undergoing arthroscopic decompression. Follow-up averaged 27 months for the open group and 20 months for the arthroscopic group, with a minimum follow-up of 1 year in both groups. Satisfactory results were obtained in 83% of the arthroscopic group and 81% of the open group using the UCLA shoulder rating scale. Patient satisfaction was 88% in the arthroscopic group compared to 94% in the open group. The higher percentage of patient satisfaction in the open group was attributable to these patients being older and less active than those of the arthroscopic group.

In 1994, Sachs and associates[30] reported results of a prospective randomized study of 41 patients followed over a 1-year period. Twenty-two patients were treated by open decompression and

19 by arthroscopic subacromial decompression. At the conclusion of 1 year, greater than 90% good and excellent results were obtained in both groups. However, over the first 3 months, the benefits of arthroscopic acromioplasty were seen. These included more rapid return of both strength and flexibility, shorter hospital stay, less narcotic usage, and a quicker return to work and daily activities. Two of the patients graded as failures in the arthroscopic group had subsequent acromioclavicular (AC) joint resections with resolution of their symptoms and returned to work. This underscores the need to evaluate the AC joint during arthroscopic subacromial decompression.

The majority of failed acromioplasties are attributable to either diagnostic errors or errors in surgical technique. Ogilvie-Harris and associates[13] in 1990 reported an evaluation of 67 shoulders in 65 patients who had continued pain and dysfunction for more than 2 years after their initial acromioplasty. In addition to a thorough history and physical examination, all these patients underwent arthroscopic evaluation. Of these 67 shoulders, 27 were felt to have failed because of diagnostic errors and 28 because of surgical errors. In only 12 had the diagnosis and procedure both been correct.

Three groups of patients with surgical errors were delineated. In five patients an AC joint resection was not performed even in the presence of AC arthritic changes. After AC joint resection, three of these obtained good results. In 12 patients, resection of bone or of the coracoacromial ligament was believed to have been inadequate. After repeat acromioplasty, six of these patients obtained a good result. Eleven additional patients formed subacromial space adhesions limiting range of motion of the shoulder. At the time of arthroscopy, these adhesions were resected and six of 11 obtained good results. Diagnoses found in this report, but not previously considered, included thoracic outlet syndrome, ulnar nerve entrapment, cervical spine pathology, osteoarthritis, labral tears, frozen shoulder, rotator cuff tear, and glenohumeral instability. One quarter of the patients who were misdiagnosed were believed to have had instability at the time of their initial operation.

Many authors have reported impingement and even partial-thickness rotator cuff tearing as a secondary event resulting from primary glenohumeral instability.[93–96] In this instance, most authors recommend correction of the primary instability without formal decompression. Our approach in these patients is to first correct the instability, most often using arthroscopic techniques. If, on preoperative evaluation, the patient is found to have a type II or type III acromial morphology, we will then perform subacromial bursoscopy. If signs of subacromial impingement are present, including undersurface acromial abrasion or bursal side partial-thickness cuff tears, we then perform subacromial decompression simply to remove the anterior lip of the acromion and to release the insertion of the coracoacromial ligament.

Like Paulos and Franklin,[15] we believe the keys to success of arthroscopic acromioplasty lie in first making an accurate diagnosis, then performing selective acromioplasty only in those patients who have failed an adequate trial of nonsurgical treatment. When acromioplasty does become necessary, it is extremely important to resect an adequate amount of bone from the undersurface and anterior aspect of the acromion, as well as to resect the insertion of the coracoacromial ligament and osteophytes present on the inferior surface of the distal clavicle. If full-thickness rotator cuff tears are encountered, we feel these should be repaired whenever possible.

ARTHROSCOPIC DISTAL CLAVICLE RESECTION

Equally acceptable results have been documented using either the direct or indirect approach to arthroscopic distal clavicle resection.[41,42,50,51,56–58] The general principles for either method remain the same. Each provides a minimally invasive technique of distal clavicle resection. When using either technique, it is extremely important to maintain the integrity of the superior AC capsule and ligamentous structures.

In 1994, Kay and associates[57] described the results of their initial ten consecutive patients at 14 months' follow-up. The patients were given UCLA shoulder rating scores postoperatively and all shoulders graded satisfactory. The greatest improvements were noted in categories of pain and function. All patients who were recreational athletes were able to return to their previous level of athletics. No complications were noted.

Tolin and Snyder[41] in 1993 reported results of 23 patients over an 18-month follow-up period. The average length of distal clavicle resection was 1.4 cm. Of these patients, 87% graded good or excellent on the UCLA shoulder rating scale, and 96% of patients were satisfied with their procedure. No complications were encountered.

In 1995, Snyder and associates[58] detailed results of a retrospective series of 50 shoulders. Follow-up averaged 2 years. Ninety-four percent of patients had satisfactory results using the UCLA shoulder score, and 98% were satisfied with their procedure. In this report, 94% of the patients had concurrent arthroscopic subacromial decompression, proving that acceptable results can be expected with a combination of these two procedures. Overall, 89% of these patients were able to return to their preinjury level of athletics. On follow-up examination, 8% of the patients had AC tenderness, 12% had palpable AC crepitus, and 4% had a positive horizontal adduction test. There were also four patients who had postoperative calcification noted at the site of distal clavicle resection. UCLA shoulder scores for these patients included two excellent, one fair, and one poor result.

Flatow and associates[42] reported initial results using the superior approach for distal clavicle resection. This study compared six open versus six arthroscopic distal clavicle resections. Follow-up averaged 30 months for the open group and 18 months for the arthroscopic group. They found comparable pain relief and function in both groups, but pain relief and return to function were achieved an average of 3.4 months earlier in the arthroscopic group. There were no complications among the arthroscopic group. Among the open group, one patient formed a keloid at his incision site and two patients complained of skin numbness. The authors concluded that, using arthroscopic techniques, satisfactory bone removal was possible with the added benefit of reduced morbidity.

Bigliani and associates[56] reported results of 42 shoulders followed up for an average of 21 months. Ninety-one percent of these patients had resolution of symptoms and returned to normal activities. Exceptional results were obtained in this series despite the removal of only 5 to 6 mm of the distal clavicle. As long as the integrity of the AC ligaments was maintained and the resection of the distal clavicle was even, this was believed to be an adequate length of resection. Two patients in this report were noted to have failed due to retained posterior cortical ridges leading to recurrence of symptoms. Results in patients treated by distal clavicle resection for previous grade II AC separation were less encouraging. Only 37% of these patients obtained satisfactory results. This was believed to be a result of persistent AC instability in this subset of patients.

The retrospective results of 41 shoulders with an average follow-up of 31 months were detailed by Flatow and associates[51] in 1995. Among those patients with diagnoses of osteoarthritis and distal clavicle osteolysis, 93% satisfactory results were obtained. Among the group with AC instability (grade II AC separation or hypermobility), however, only 58% satisfactory results were obtained. This was a confirmation of the results reported by Bigliani and associates[56] and it was proposed that in this subset of patients a distal clavicle resection should not be performed alone, but rather in conjunction with an AC stabilization procedure. One patient within this group was revised arthroscopically for an uneven resection and four additional patients underwent AC stabilization procedures.

Overall, the results of arthroscopic distal clavicle resection, if performed properly, have proven superior to those of open distal clavicle resection. Reported unsuccessful results have been due to abutment of the distal clavicle on the acromion, postoperative instability of the AC joint, or uneven resection with a retained cortical rim of the distal clavicle.[42,51,56] Postoperative acromioclavicular abutment is believed to result more from destabilization of the AC joint than from an inadequate bony resection.[51] This underscores the importance of achieving a smooth bony resection, as well as preserving the AC capsular structures. If the integrity of these structures is violated during the course of the operation, the AC joint will be rendered unstable. In this instance, we feel it appropriate to make a small superior incision and perform an AC stabilization procedure to avoid future complications.

ROTATOR CUFF REPAIR

We believe the ultimate goal of surgery should be to obtain a water-tight closure of the rotator cuff and to restore the functional integrity of the tendons. Although some studies have documented a poor correlation between integrity of the rotator cuff and functional outcome,[72,73,97] other authors have disputed these findings.[98,99] In reports by Liu and Baker,[72–74] the integrity of the cuff depended on the original tear size, with large tears having a significantly higher percentage of postoperative rotator cuff defects. These studies, however, could find no significant correlation between functional outcome and postoperative rotator cuff integrity.

Lundberg[98] described arthrogram-confirmed postoperative full-thickness rotator cuff tears in seven of 21 patients. These seven were noted to be significantly more symptomatic than those with negative arthrograms. Harryman and associates[99] in 1991 documented better functional outcomes in those patients who had intact rotator cuff repairs. Although correlation between rotator cuff integrity and functional outcome is questionable, our goal in each rotator cuff repair is to achieve closure of the defect and to improve functional outcome.

Arthroscopic Rotator Cuff Repair

The results of arthroscopic rotator cuff repair are still evolving. In 1996, JW Tippett (personal communication, Atlanta, GA, 1996) reported results of 29 patients with an average follow-up of 16 months. He found 21 of 29 satisfactory results using a modified UCLA scale. Complications were not included. In 1995, EM Wolf (personal communication, San Antonio, TX, 1995) reported 85% good and excellent results in 66 patients who underwent arthroscopic rotator cuff repair.

He stated that 92% of these patients were satisfied with the procedure. The length of follow-up was not mentioned.

Stollsteimer and Savoie[76] reported the results of 48 patients who underwent arthroscopic repair of full-thickness rotator cuff defects. Average follow-up in this group of patients was 34 months, with a minimum follow-up of 12 months. Twenty-seven repairs were performed by transtendon techniques, and 21 were performed with suture passing techniques. The patients were evaluated based on UCLA scores. The scores for all patients averaged 33 out of a possible 35. No significant difference was found when assessing functional outcome based on size of the tear. Patients were also grouped by age, and again no significant difference in functional outcome was noted. One failure was documented. This was a repeat rupture of the rotator cuff in a 40-year-old man. The patient underwent open revision repair of his rotator cuff and has done well.

Mini-Open Rotator Cuff Repair

Arthroscopic assisted techniques of rotator cuff repair have produced results equivalent or superior to those of standard open rotator cuff repair. Levy and associates[66] in 1990 reported results of 25 patients undergoing arthroscopic assisted rotator cuff repair. Average follow-up was 18 months, with a minimum 12-month follow-up. Eighty percent good and excellent results were achieved using the UCLA shoulder rating scale; 96% of patients were satisfied. Among those patients with small and moderate sized rotator cuff tears, 100% satisfaction was obtained. Among those patients with large and massive tears, however, 71% satisfactory rates were obtained. This would seem to imply this technique is more appropriate for small and moderate sized rotator cuff tears.

In 1994, Liu[73] reported results of 44 patients with a 4.2-year average follow-up. He reported 84% good and excellent results using the UCLA shoulder rating scale, and 88% of patients were satisfied with their result. When looking specifically at athletes, 64% were able to return to sports at their previous level of competition. If only those athletes with small and moderate tears were considered, 80% were able to return to their previous levels of competition. Complications in this series included two postoperative frozen shoulders, one superficial wound infection, two cases of impingement syndrome, and no apparent rerupture.

In 1994, Paulos and Kody[75] reported results of 18 patients with an average follow-up of 46 months and a minimum follow-up of 36 months. Eighty-eight percent good and excellent results were obtained with a 94% rate of satisfaction among patients. Only two complications were encountered in their series, a superficial infection and a failed repair.

Results of a comparison study of open versus arthroscopically assisted rotator cuff repairs were reported by Baker and Liu.[72] This was a retrospective review of 20 shoulders repaired in an open fashion versus 17 shoulders repaired in an arthroscopically assisted fashion. Follow-up was 3.3 years for the open group versus 3.2 years for the arthroscopically assisted group. The UCLA rating scale was used for functional evaluation with 80% good and excellent results reported for the open group versus 85% good and excellent results for the arthroscopically assisted group. Rates of patient satisfaction were 88% for the open group versus 92% for the arthroscopically assisted group. Return to activity was approximately 1 month shorter in the arthroscopically assisted group at 4.5 months total. They concluded that small and moderate sized rotator cuff tears had a better functional outcome after arthroscopically assisted rotator cuff repair, and that this was as effective as open repair for the treatment of rotator cuff defects.

Open Rotator Cuff Repair

Many authors have reported good results with open rotator cuff repair.[67–71] Most reports indicate that failure of open rotator cuff repair has been caused by long-term weakness, denervation of the deltoid, or deltoid retraction.[66] The techniques previously described should theoretically eliminate the majority of these complications. When performing our modification of the open rotator cuff repair, the deltoid is always repaired in the manner described. This repair is quite secure and our postoperative protocol is not modified. We have had no episodes of deltoid dehiscence using this technique.

CONCLUSION

Advances in arthroscopic surgery have increased the knowledge of rotator cuff disease. We can now evaluate and treat the various stages of rotator cuff disease using minimally invasive techniques. Although these techniques are technically demanding, appropriately applied they offer several advantages over traditional open procedures. Arthroscopic acromioplasty and arthroscopic distal clavicle resection have produced satisfactory long-term results. Arthroscopic rotator cuff repair techniques are in their early stages and further long-term studies are indicated. Mini-open rotator cuff repair techniques have documented success rates equal to those of open rotator cuff repair.

REFERENCES

1. Imhoff A, Ledermann T: Arthroscopic subacromial decompression with and without the Holmium: YAG-laser. A prospective comparative study. *Arthroscopy* 1995;11:549–556.

2. Bigliani LU, Morrison DS, April EW: The morphology of the acromion and its relationship to rotator cuff tears. *Orthop Trans* 1986;10:228.

3. Ellman H, Harris E, Kay SP: Early degenerative joint disease simulating impingement syndrome: Arthroscopic findings. *Arthroscopy* 1992;8:482–487.

4. Fu FH, Harner CD, Klein AH: Shoulder impingement syndrome: A critical review. *Clin Orthop* 1991;269:162–173.

5. Hawkins RJ, Kennedy JC: Impingement syndrome in athletes. *Am J Sports Med* 1980;8:151–158.

6. Liu SH, Boynton E: Posterior superior impingement of the rotator cuff on the glenoid rim as a cause of shoulder pain in the overhead athlete. *Arthroscopy* 1993;9:697–699.

7. Nirschl RP: Rotator cuff tendinitis: Basic concepts of pathoetiology, in Barr JS Jr (ed): *Instructional Course Lectures XXXVIII*. Park Ridge, IL, American Academy of Orthopaedic Surgeons, 1989, pp 439–445.

8. Rathbun JB, Macnab I: The microvascular pattern of the rotator cuff. *J Bone Joint Surg* 1970;52B:540–553.

9. Neer CS II: Anterior acromioplasty for the chronic impingement syndrome in the shoulder: A preliminary report. *J Bone Joint Surg* 1972;54A:41–50.

10. Neer CS II: Impingement lesions. *Clin Orthop* 1983;173:70–77.

11. Jobe FW: Impingement problems in the athlete, in Barr JS Jr (ed): *Instructional Course Lectures XXXVIII*. Park Ridge, IL, American Academy of Orthopaedic Surgeons, 1989, pp 205–209.

12. Ellman H: Arthroscopic treatment of impingement of the shoulder, in Barr JS Jr (ed): *Instructional Course Lectures XXXVIII*. Park Ridge, IL, American Academy of Orthopaedic Surgeons, 1989, pp 177–185.

13. Ogilvie-Harris DJ, Wiley AM, Sattarian J: Failed acromioplasty for impingement syndrome. *J Bone Joint Surg* 1990;72B:1070–1072.

14. Altchek DW, Warren RF, Wickiewicz TL, Skyhar MJ, Ortiz G, Schwartz E: Arthroscopic acromioplasty: Technique and results. *J Bone Joint Surg* 1990;72A:1198–1207.

15. Paulos LE, Franklin JL: Arthroscopic shoulder decompression development and application: A five year experience. *Am J Sports Med* 1990;18:235–244.

16. Morrison DS, Bigliani LU: Variations in acromial shape and its effect on rotator cuff tears, in Takagishi N (ed): *The Shoulder*. Tokyo, Japan, Professional Post Graduate Services, 1987, pp 213–214.

17. Penny JN, Welsh RP: Shoulder impingement syndromes in athletes and their surgical management. *Am J Sports Med* 1981;9:11–15.

18. Post M, Cohen J: Impingement syndrome: A review of late stage II and early stage III lesions. *Clin Orthop* 1986;207:126–132.

19. Tibone JE, Jobe FW, Kerlan RK, et al: Shoulder impingement syndrome in athletes treated by an anterior acromioplasty. *Clin Orthop* 1985;198:134–140.

20. Ellman H: Arthroscopic subacromial decompression: Analysis of one- to three-year results. *Arthroscopy* 1987;3:173–181.

21. Gartsman GM, Blair ME Jr, Noble PC, Bennett JB, Tullos HS: Arthroscopic subacromial decompression: An anatomical study. *Am J Sports Med* 1988;16:48–50.

22. Burns TP, Turba JE: Arthroscopic treatment of shoulder impingement in athletes. *Am J Sports Med* 1992;20:13–16.

23. Ellman H, Kay SP: Arthroscopic subacromial decompression for chronic impingement: Two- to five-year results. *J Bone Joint Surg* 1991;73B:395–398.

24. Gartsman GM: Arthroscopic acromioplasty for lesions of the rotator cuff. *J Bone Joint Surg* 1990;72A:169–180.

25. Roye RP, Grana WA, Yates CK: Arthroscopic subacromial decompression: Two- to seven-year follow-up. *Arthroscopy* 1995;11:301–306.

26. Speer KP, Lohnes J, Garrett WE Jr: Arthroscopic subacromial decompression: Results in advanced impingement syndrome. *Arthroscopy* 1991;7:291–296.

27. Ryu RK: Arthroscopic subacromial decompression: A clinical review. *Arthroscopy* 1992;8:141–147.

28. Van Holsbeeck E, DeRycke J, Declercq G, Martens M, Verstreken J, Fabry G: Subacromial impingement: Open versus arthroscopic decompression. *Arthroscopy* 1992;8:173–178.

29. Norlin R: Arthroscopic subacromial decompression versus open acromioplasty. *Arthroscopy* 1989;5:321–323.

30. Sachs RA, Stone ML, Devine S: Open versus arthroscopic acromioplasty: A prospective randomized study. *Arthroscopy* 1994;10:248–254.

31. Lazarus MD, Chansky HA, Misra S, Williams GR, Iannotti JP: Comparison of open and arthroscopic subacromial decompression. *J Shoulder Elbow Surg* 1994;3:1–11.

32. Caspari RB, Thal R: A Technique for arthroscopic subacromial decompression. *Arthroscopy* 1992;8:23–30.

33. Caspari RB, Thal R: Arthroscopic subacromial decompression: Technical considerations. *Tech Orthop* 1994;9:102–107.

34. Sampson TG, Nisbet JK, Glick JM: Precision acromioplasty in arthroscopic subacromial decompression of the shoulder. *Arthroscopy* 1991;7:301–307.

35. Warren JJ, Kann S, Maddox LM: The "Arthroscopic Impingement Test." *Arthroscopy* 1994;10:224–230.

36. Morrison DS, Schaefer RK, Friedman RL: The relationship between subacromial space pressure, blood pressure, and visual clarity during arthroscopic subacromial decompression. *Arthroscopy* 1995;11:557–560.

37. Ogilvie-Harris DJ, Boynton E: Arthroscopic acromioplasty: Extravasation of fluid into the deltoid muscle. *Arthroscopy* 1990;6:52–54.

38. Beach WR, Caspari RB: Arthroscopic management of rotator cuff disease. *Orthopedics* 1993;16:1007–1015.

39. Miller C, Savoie FH: Glenohumeral abnormalities associated with full-thickness tears of the rotator cuff. *Orthop Rev* 1994;23:159–162.

40. Gartsman GM: Arthroscopic treatment of rotator cuff disease. *J Shoulder Elbow Surg* 1995; 4:228–241.

41. Tolin BS, Snyder SJ: Our technique for the arthroscopic Mumford procedure. *Orthop Clin North Am* 1993;24:143–151.

42. Flatow EL, Cordasco FA, Bigliani LU: Arthroscopic resection of the outer end of the clavicle from a superior approach: A critical, quantitative, radiographic assessment of bone removal. *Arthroscopy* 1992;8:55–64.

43. Mumford EB: Acromioclavicular dislocation: A new operative treatment. *J Bone Joint Surg* 1941;23A:799–802.

44. Gurd FB: The treatment of complete dislocation of the outer end of the clavicle: An hitherto undescribed operation. *Ann Surg* 1941; 113:1094–1098.

45. Petersson CJ: Resection of the lateral end of the clavicle: A 3- to 30-year follow-up. *Acta Orthop Scand* 1983;54:904–907.

46. Rockwood CA Jr, Young DC: Disorders of the acromioclavicular joint, in Rockwood CA Jr, Matsen FA III (eds): *The Shoulder.* Philadelphia, PA, WB Saunders, 1990, pp 413–476.

47. Taft TN, Wilson FC, Oglesby JW: Dislocation of the acromioclavicular joint: An end-result study. *J Bone Joint Surg* 1987;69A:1045–1051.

48. Pattee GA, Snyder SJ: Synovial chondromatosis of the acromioclavicular joint: A case report. *Clin Orthop* 1988;233:205–207.

49. Cook FF, Tibone JE: The Mumford procedure in athletes: An objective analysis of function. *Am J Sports Med* 1988;16:97–100.

50. Gartsman GM, Combs AH, Davis PF, Tullos HS: Arthroscopic acromioclavicular joint resection: An anatomical study. *Am J Sports Med* 1991;19:2–5.

51. Flatow EL, Duralde XA, Nicholson GP, Pollock RG, Bigliani LU: Arthroscopic resection of the distal clavicle with a superior approach. *J Shoulder Elbow Surg* 1995;4:41–50.

52. Blazar PE, Iannotti JP, Williams GR: Anteroposterior instability of the clavicle after distal clavicle resection. *Clin Orthop,* in press.

53. Daluga DJ, Dobozi W: The Influence of distal clavicle resection and rotator cuff repair on the effectiveness of anterior acromioplasty. *Clin Orthop* 1989;247:117–123.

54. Walsh WM, Peterson DA, Shelton G, Neumann RD: Shoulder strength following acromioclavicular injury. *Am J Sports Med* 1985;13:153–158.

55. Esch JC, Ozerkis LR, Helgager JA, Kane N, Lilliott N: Arthroscopic subacromial decompression: Results according to the degree of rotator cuff tear. *Arthroscopy* 1988;4:241–249.

56. Bigliani LU, Nicholson GP, Flatow EL: Arthroscopic resection of the distal clavicle. Orthop *Clin North Am* 1993;24:133–141.

57. Kay SP, Ellman H, Harris E: Arthroscopic distal clavicle excision: Technique and early results. *Clin Orthop* 1994;301:181–184.

58. Snyder SJ, Banas MP, Karzel RP: The arthroscopic Mumford procedure: An analysis of results. *Arthroscopy* 1995;11:157–164.

59. Fukuda K, Craig EV, An KN, Cofield RH, Chao EY: Biomechanical study of the ligamentous system of the acromioclavicular joint. *J Bone Joint Surg* 1986;68A:434–440.

60. Klimkiewicz J, Williams GR, Sher J, Karduna A, DeJardins J, Iannotti JP: The acromioclavicular capsule as a restraint to posterior translation of the clavicle. *J Shoulder Elbow Surg,* in press.

61. Burkhart SS: Arthroscopic treatment of massive rotator cuff tears: Clinical results and biomechanical rationale. *Orthop Trans* 1990;14:173.

62. Rockwood CA Jr, Burkhead WZ: Management of patients with massive rotator cuff defects by acromioplasty and rotator cuff debridement. *Orthop Trans* 1988;12:190–191.

63. Levy HJ, Gardner RD, Lemak LJ: Arthroscopic subacromial decompression in the treatment of full-thickness rotator cuff tears. *Arthroscopy* 1991;7:8–13.

64. Hawkins RJ, Misamore GW, Hobeika PE: Surgery for full-thickness rotator-cuff tears. *J Bone Joint Surg* 1985;67A:1349–1355.

65. Montgomery TJ, Yerger B, Savoie FH III: Management of rotator cuff tears: A comparison of arthroscopic debridement and surgical repair. *J Shoulder Elbow Surg* 1994;3:70–78.

66. Levy HJ, Uribe JW, Delaney LG: Arthroscopic assisted rotator cuff repair: Preliminary results. *Arthroscopy* 1990;6:55–60.

67. Bigliani LU, McIlveen SJ, Cordasco F, Musso E: Operative repair of massive rotator cuff tears: Long term results. *Orthop Trans* 1990;14:251.

68. Cofield RH, Hoffmeyer P, Lanzer WL: Surgical repair of chronic rotator cuff tears. *Orthop Trans* 1990;14:251–252.

69. Ellman H, Hanker G, Bayer M: Repair of the rotator cuff: End-result study of factors influencing reconstruction. *J Bone Joint Surg* 1986;68A:1136–1144.

70. Neer CS II, Flatow EL, Lech O: Tears of the rotator cuff: Long term results of anterior acromioplasty and repair. *Orthop Trans* 1988;12:735.

71. Post M, Silver R, Singh M: Rotator cuff tear: Diagnosis and treatment. *Clin Orthop* 1983; 173:78–91.

72. Baker CL, Liu SH: Comparison of open and arthroscopically assisted rotator cuff repairs. *Am J Sports Med* 1995;23:99–104.

73. Liu SH: Arthroscopically-assisted rotator-cuff repair. *J Bone Joint Surg* 1994;76B:592–595.

74. Liu SH, Baker CL: Arthroscopically assisted rotator cuff repair: Correlation of functional results with integrity of the cuff. *Arthroscopy* 1994;10:54–60.

75. Paulos LE, Kody MH: Arthroscopically enhanced "mini-approach" to rotator cuff repair. *Am J Sports Med* 1994;22:19–25.

76. Stollsteimer GT, Savoie FH III: Arthroscopic rotator cuff repair: Current indications, limitations, techniques, and results, in Cannon WD (ed): *Instructional Course Lectures 47.* Rosemont, IL, American Academy of Orthopaedic Surgeons, in press.

77. Brems J: Rotator cuff tear: Evaluation and treatment. *Orthopedics* 1988;11:69–81.

78. Zvijac JE, Levy HJ, Lemak LJ: Arthroscopic subacromial decompression in the treatment of full thickness rotator cuff tears: A 3 to 6-year follow-up. *Arthroscopy* 1994;10:518–523.

79. DePalma AF (ed): *Degenerative Changes in the Sternoclavicular and Acromioclavicular Joints in Various Decades.* Springfield, IL, CC Thomas, 1957.

80. Petersson CJ, Redlund-Johnell I: Radiographic joint space in normal acromioclavicular joints. *Acta Orthop Scand* 1983;54:431–433.

81. Watson M: The refractory painful arc syndrome. *J Bone Joint Surg* 1978;60B:544–546.

82. Neviaser TJ, Neviaser RJ, Neviaser JS, Neviaser JS. The four-in-one arthroplasty for the painful arc syndrome. *Clin Orthop* 1982;163:107–112.

83. Olsewski JM, Depew AD: Arthroscopic subacromial decompression and rotator cuff debridement for stage II and stage III impingement. *Arthroscopy* 1994;10:61–68.

84. Johnson LL (ed): *Arthroscopic Surgery: Principles in Practice,* ed 3. St. Louis, MO, CV Mosby, 1986, vol 2, pp 1301–1445.

85. Meyers JF: Arthroscopic debridement of the acromioclavicular joint and distal clavicle resection, in McGinty JB, Caspari RB, Jackson RW, Poehling GG (eds): *Operative Arthroscopy*. New York, NY, Raven Press, 1991, pp 557–560.

86. Hecker AT, Shea M, Hayhurst JO, Myers ER, Meeks LW, Hayes WC: Pull-out strength of suture anchors for rotator cuff and Bankart lesion repairs. *Am J Sports Med* 1993;21:874–879.

87. Reed SC, Glossop N, Ogilvie-Harris DJ: Full-thickness rotator cuff tears: A biomechanical comparison of suture versus bone anchor techniques. *Am J Sports Med* 1996;24:46–48.

88. Burkhart SS: The Deadman Theory of suture anchors: Observations along a south Texas fence line. *Arthroscopy* 1995;11:119–123.

89. Gerber C, Schneeberger AG, Beck M, Schlegel U: Mechanical strength of repairs of the rotator cuff. *J Bone Joint Surg* 1994;76B:371–380.

90. Snyder SJ: Evaluation and treatment of the rotator cuff. *Orthop Clin North Am* 1993;24:173–192.

91. Burkhart SS: Reconciling the paradox of rotator cuff repair versus debridement: A unified biomechanic rationale for the treatment of rotator cuff tears. *Arthroscopy* 1994;10:4–19.

92. Snyder SJ, Pachelli AF, Del Pizzo W, Friedman MJ, Ferkel RD, Pattee G: Partial thickness rotator cuff tears: Results of arthroscopic treatment. *Arthroscopy* 1991;7:1–7.

93. Warren RF: Subluxation of the shoulder in athletes. *Clin Sports Med* 1983;2:339–354.

94. Garth WP Jr, Allman FL Jr, Armstrong WS: Occult anterior subluxations of the shoulder in noncontact sports. *Am J Sports Med* 1987;15:579–585.

95. Jobe FW, Kvitne RS, Giangarra CE: Shoulder pain in the overhand or throwing athlete: The relationship of anterior instability and rotator cuff impingement. *Orthop Rev* 1989;18:963–975.

96. Glasgow SG, Bruce RA, Yacobucci GN, Torg JS: Arthroscopic resection of glenoid labral tears in the athlete: A report of 29 cases. *Arthroscopy* 1992;8:48–54.

97. Calvert PT, Packer NP, Stoker DJ, Bayley JI, Kessel L: Arthrography of the shoulder after operative repair of the torn rotator cuff. *J Bone Joint Surg* 1986;68B:147–150.

98. Lundberg BJ: The correlation of clinical evaluation with operative findings and prognosis in rotator cuff rupture, in Bayley I, Kessel L (eds): *Shoulder Surgery*. Berlin, Germany, Springer-Verlag, 1982, pp 35–38.

99. Harryman DT II, Mack LA, Wang KY, Jackins SE, Richardson ML, Matsen FA III: Repairs of the rotator cuff: Correlation of functional results with integrity of the cuff. *J Bone Joint Surg* 1991;73A:982–989.

TREATMENT OF MASSIVE ROTATOR CUFF TEARS: POSTERIOR-SUPERIOR AND ANTERIOR-SUPERIOR

JON J.P. WARNER, MD

CHRISTIAN GERBER, MD

The purpose of this chapter is to consider treatment approaches to massive rotator cuff tears of two different anatomic configurations. Tears that involve the supraspinatus, infraspinatus, and teres minor are termed posterior-superior tears, whereas tears that involve the subscapularis and supraspinatus are termed anterior-superior tears. The distinction between these two patterns of injury is important, because the epidemiology, mechanism of injury, disability, and prognosis differ.

All clinical decisions must be made in the context of a sound understanding of relevant functional anatomy, biomechanics, and natural history of these types of rotator cuff tears. The specific treatment pitfalls in diagnosis and management of these conditions will be presented. Patient selection and deselection for reconstructive and salvage procedures will also be addressed.

Massive posterior-superior rotator cuff tears comprise only a small percentage of all tears. In Neer's series[1] of 340 rotator cuff tears operated on over a 13-year period, 145 were classified as massive. Bigliani and associates[2] operated on 61 massive rotator cuff tears over a 6-year period; and over a 12-year period, Ellman and associates[3] performed 50 rotator cuff tear repairs, of which nine (18%) were massive. Harryman and associates[4] reviewed 105 cases, of which 28 had a tear involving both the supraspinatus and infraspinatus, and an additional 22 also involved the subscapularis. Finally, Hawkins and associates[5] reported that of 100 consecutive cases over a 5-year period, 27 were massive rotator cuff tears. One author (CG) operated on a series of 50 massive rotator cuff tears over a 3-year period, while the other author (JPW) has surgically treated 53 massive rotator cuff tears out of 213 rotator cuff tears during a 5-year period.

There is no universal agreement on the definition of massive rotator cuff tears.[6–8] In North America, Cofield's definition[9] generally is applied, with a massive tear having a maximum diameter of greater than 5 cm. Clinical studies done by experienced shoulder surgeons have led to the determination that tissue quality is at least as important as tear size in determining the potential for a secure surgical repair. For example, an acute, massive tear may be much larger than 5 cm in diameter but have robust, elastic tendon tissue that easily is repaired to its anatomic insertion, whereas a chronic, smaller tear may have thin, friable, inelastic tendon tissue that mobilizes poorly and is repaired only tenuously.

It is our preference to measure the extent of disinsertion of the cuff after trimming away the degenerated rim of tissue.[7] Because arm position may determine the appearance of tear diameter, the dimension of the detached cuff is measured in centimeters when the arm is at the side, and the tear is further defined by how many tendons are involved. Thus, a more functional definition of massive tear, rather than simply expressing the maximum diameter of the tendon tear, is one involving two or more tendons.

Any surgeon faced with treating a massive rotator cuff tear must be self-critical about patient selection, surgical treatment, and ultimate functional outcome. This approach is necessary if the benefits of surgery are to be realistically expressed to the patient. The natural history of surgical treatment of these kinds of tears is good pain relief but some moderate to severe residual weakness. Most patients will have some degree of limitation of upper extremity endurance for work and sport activities. If this expectation is considered, it is possible to develop an awareness of the potential pitfalls in patient selection and treatment.

Although successful tendon healing is not always directly correlated with a good clinical outcome, powerful shoulder function usually requires an intact tendon repair. In general, the surgeon may anticipate some improvement in function as well as pain, if the preoperative, surgical, and post-operative rehabilitation plans are well formulated and executed in each individual patient situation.

PREOPERATIVE CONSIDERATIONS

We believe each treatment plan must be formulated on an individualized basis. The overall disability of the patient should be considered in the context of his or her pain. Coexistent medical conditions may be a contraindication for an aggressive reconstructive approach because of higher morbidity or mortality. An example would be an elderly, frail, female patient with cardiac problems. This kind of patient might be more safely treated with a less aggressive approach than an otherwise healthy 50-year-old male, even though they have similar rotator cuff pathology (ie, similar size tear). Moreover, these patients will have different functional needs and goals. The elderly female might have more of a problem with pain and need functional recovery only for activities of daily living, whereas the healthy male might also require strength for forceful overhead activities or sports.

PATHOANATOMY AND PATHOMECHANICS

SIZE OF THE TENDON TEAR

The force potential of a muscle is determined based on its physiologic cross-sectional area (PCSA).[10] A muscle's leverage is determined based on a perpendicular drawn from its line of action to the center of rotation of the humeral head.[11] If a muscle's force potential is multiplied by its leverage, its functional contribution to joint rotation can be determined. An analysis of the rotator cuff muscles demonstrates that the supraspinatus has a relatively small PCSA and its

rotational potential for abduction is only 14% compared to the other muscles of the rotator cuff.[10,11] Its smaller size and closer insertion to the axis of rotation of the joint is the reason for this low rotational potential, although its mechanical advantage is greatest in the first 30° of abduction. Therefore, the supraspinatus is more important in initiating abduction. Conversely, the infraspinatus/teres minor and subscapularis have a rotational potential during abduction of 32% and 52%, respectively.[10]

During simple scapular plane abduction, the tendon excursions of the rotator cuff muscles are small (range 0.5 to 4.0 cm) compared to those of the deltoid muscle (6.5 cm);[12] therefore, they function more as stabilizers, which provide a fixed fulcrum for concentric rotation of the humeral head on the glenoid, than as prime movers.[13,14] During early abduction, the deltoid creates a relative upward shearing moment that must be resisted by a force couple with the combined rotator cuff muscles. Disruption of the rotator cuff weakens the stabilizing effect that resists this superior translation.[15–18] The posterior (infraspinatus/teres minor) and anterior (subscapularis) rotator cuff muscles are very important for this force couple. The long head of the biceps brachii also resists anterior and superior translation of the humeral head on the glenoid,[19–21] and this structure is often noted to be enlarged or "hypertrophied" in patients with large rotator cuff tears.[1]

Clinical[22–24] and experimental observations[25] have shown that even large tears of the rotator cuff can be consistent with good motion and concentric rotation of the glenohumeral joint (Fig. 33). These types of patients will have a tendon tear that is large and involves the entire supraspinatus, but little of the subscapularis or infraspinatus. It is extension of the tear into the anterior or posterior cuff tendons that results in loss of containment and superior translation of the humeral head.[7,22,23,26] Conversely, some patients with a small or large rotator cuff tear may have poor function (Fig. 33, B). This understanding that size of the tear does not always correlate precisely with function helps explain the disparity of experience in surgical treatment of

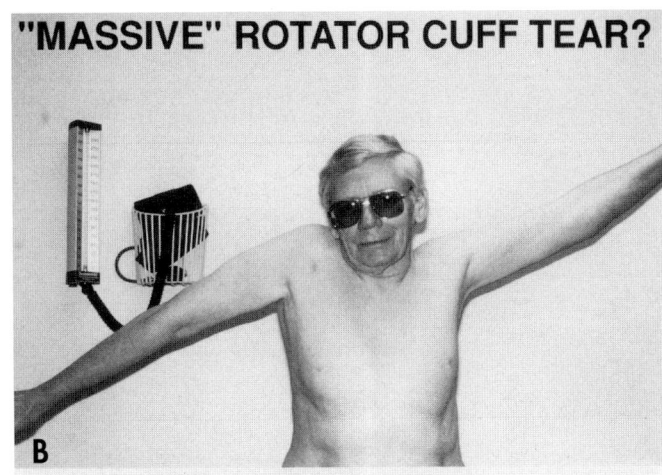

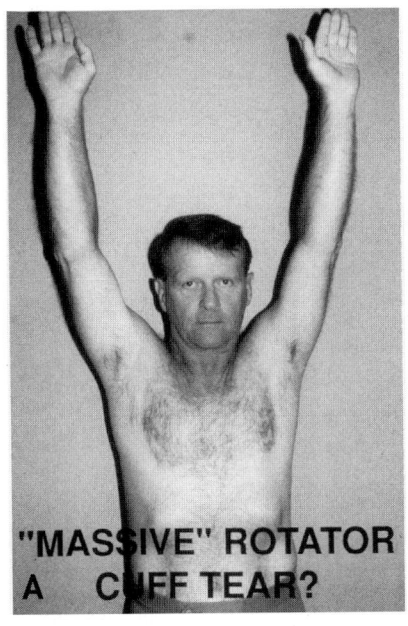

FIGURE 33
A, 58-year-old man with bilateral massive rotator cuff tears and good function following only arthroscopic debridement.
B, 62-year-old man with chronic massive right rotator cuff tear involving the supraspinatus and infraspinatus tendons.
(Reproduced with permission from Warner JJP, Gerber C: Massive tears of the posterior-superior rotator cuff, in Warner JJP, Iannotti JP, Gerber C (eds): *Complex and Revision Problems in Shoulder Surgery.* Philadelphia, PA, Lippincott-Raven, 1997, pp 177–202.)

massive rotator cuff tears that can be found in the literature.[2,3,6-9,22-24,26-40] This disparity is probably related to the degree of atrophy and fatty degeneration of the muscles of the rotator cuff.[17]

ROLE OF MUSCLE ATROPHY AND FATTY DEGENERATION

The term "massive rotator cuff tear" describes a heterogeneous population of patients with varying degrees of shoulder dysfunction. Overall shoulder function and external rotation weakness can be directly correlated with the degree of fatty atrophy of the infraspinatus muscle in patients with massive rotator cuff tears involving the posterior cuff.[39,40] Moreover, such changes may predict the quality of tendon tissue at the time of surgery. For example, a patient with an acute rotator cuff tear and a magnetic resonance imaging scan (MRI) that demonstrates a homogeneous and large muscle will have tendon tissue that is robust and elastic. Conversely, a patient with a chronic rotator cuff tear and an MRI that demonstrates an atrophied muscle, which is heterogeneous with the appearance of intramuscular fat, will have a tendon that is inelastic and friable (Gerber, personal communication). Such muscle changes may be chronic and irreversible following surgery[41] (Fig. 34).

ROLE OF THE CORACOACROMIAL ARCH

This structure has an important secondary stabilizing role in which it prevents anterior-superior translation in cases where the rotator cuff containment function is lost.[27,42,43] In these situations, it acts as a last barrier to unchecked anterior-superior translation of the humeral head, and it

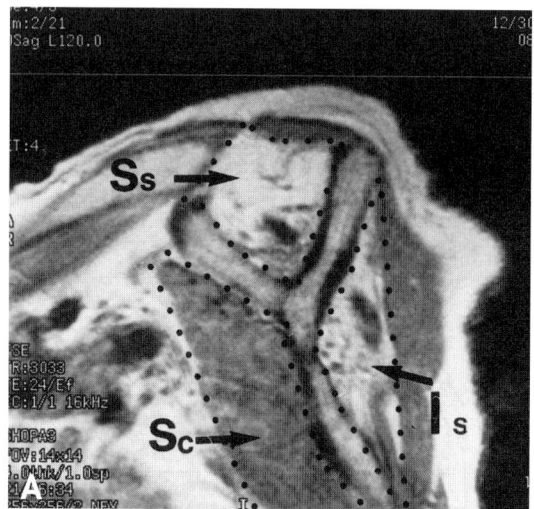 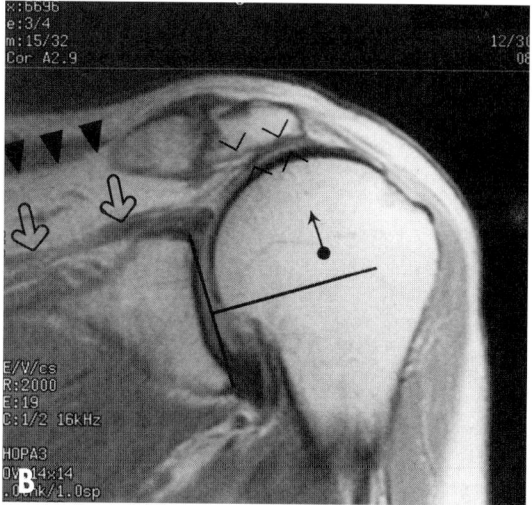

FIGURE 34

A, Oblique-sagittal magnetic resonance image (MRI) for a 68-year-old man with chronic massive tear of the supraspinatus and infraspinatus of the left shoulder. Note complete fatty replacement of the supraspinatus (Ss) and Infraspinatus (Is), compared to the normal subscapularis (Sc). **B,** Coronal MRI image of same patient demonstrates atrophy of the supraspinatus (large open arrows) and marked superior displacement of the humeral head (solid arrows). Note that the center of the humeral head (solid circle) is 5 mm above a line drawn perpendicular to the equator of the glenoid. The humeral head and acromion are in contact (open arrows).

must be preserved.[27] In fact, there is some debate that the type III (hooked) acromion shape may be a compensatory phenomenon that is attempting to reduce superior humeral head displacement in cases of massive rotator cuff tears. Thus, routine acromioplasty may be biomechanically inadvisable in cases of chronic, long-standing massive rotator cuff tears (Fig. 35).

BIOMECHANICS AS A RATIONALE FOR SURGICAL TREATMENT

In clinical practice, the amount of muscle atrophy on MRI and the acromiohumeral interval (AHI) on plain radiographs are very important preoperative considerations in deciding the course of treatment[3,18] (Fig. 34). If the AHI on a true anteroposterior (AP) radiograph with the arm in neutral rotation is less than 5 mm, and if there is marked muscle atrophy and fatty degeneration on the MRI, then the quality of the tendon tissue will be poor, the surgical repair of the rotator cuff will not recenter the humeral head in the glenoid, and restoration of strength and function is unlikely.[44] Conversely, a patient with only minimal superior

translation (AHI > 5 mm) and homogeneous and large rotator muscles on MRI will likely have good quality tendon tissue that can be repaired securely.

POSTERIOR-SUPERIOR ROTATOR CUFF TEARS: SUPRA- AND INFRASPINATUS ETIOLOGY

This most common configuration of rotator cuff tears typically occurs in individuals in their sixth through eighth decades of life. It is believed that, although the exact etiology of full-thickness rotator cuff tears remains a subject of debate, a gradual attrition of the tendons from "outlet impingement" results in a degenerative tear in a region with a paucity of blood supply.[1,45–47] Age-related intrinsic degeneration in the rotator cuff also probably reduces its structural strength, thus rendering it at greater risk for failure even with trivial trauma.[48] In these kinds of patients some predictions can be made about the size of the tendon tear and quality of tendon tissue based on the history given by the patient. A patient in the sixth or seventh decade of life who reports an onset of insidious pain and loss of function over a period

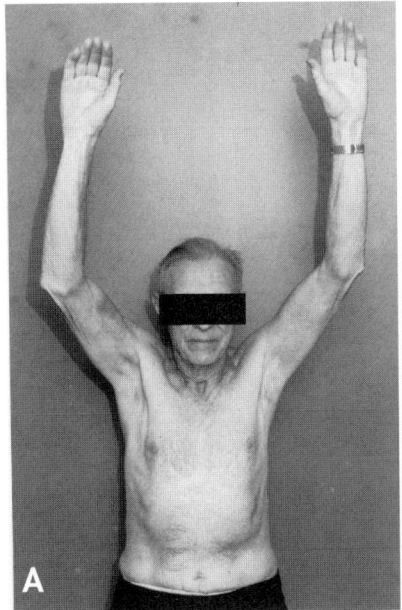
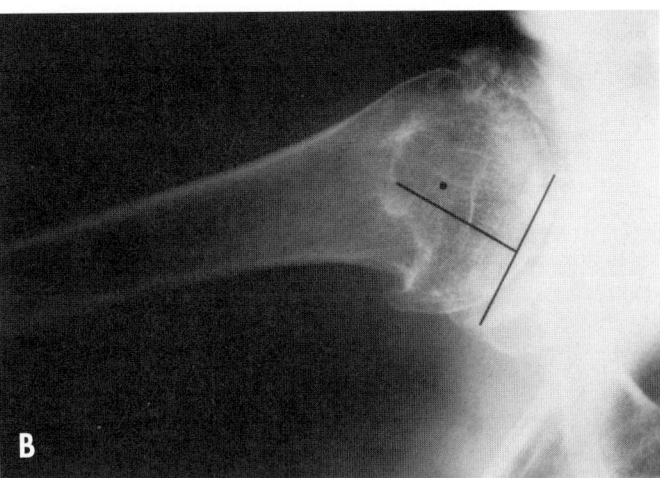

FIGURE 35

A, 78-year-old man with chronic, massive rotator cuff tear and mild pain. He plays tennis 5 days each week. **B,** True antero-posterior radiograph demonstrates arthritis and superior displacement of the humeral head. There are adaptive changes on the acromion from chronic compression. This man has well compensated function with the coracoacromial arch maintaining a fulcrum for glenohumeral rotation.

of time without any prior history of trauma is likely to have a massive posterior-superior rotator cuff tear. This kind of patient is also likely to have an MRI that shows significant atrophy and fatty degeneration of the spinati musculature.[17,41] Chronic, massive rotator cuff tears with thin, friable tendon tissue have also been associated with patients who have had multiple steroid injections or a history of chronic smoking. In these kinds of patients there is actual tendon involution or loss, and the remaining muscle and tendon are inelastic as a result of scarring and fatty degeneration[7,26] (Fig. 36). Surgical mobilization of the tendons for repair can be very difficult in these cases.[3,28] Patients with chronic, massive rotator cuff tears may also develop disuse osteopenia of the proximal humerus, which can make secure tendon-bone repair more difficult to achieve.

A different kind of patient is one in the fifth or six decade who reports a specific traumatic event preceding the onset of shoulder pain and poor

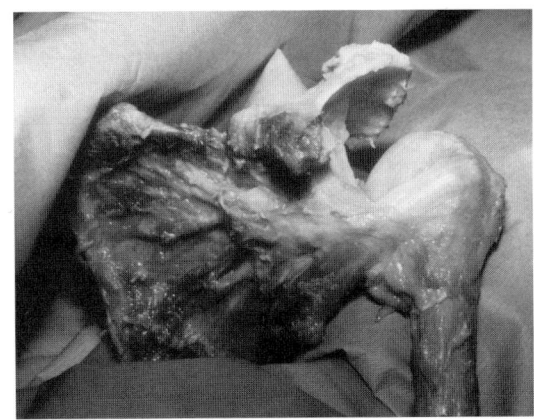

FIGURE 36

Cadaveric shoulder of a 78-year-old man with chronic massive rotator cuff tear. There is loss of tendon substance of the supraspinatus and infraspinatus, and corresponding muscle loss as well. (Reproduced with permission from Warner JJP, Gerber C: Massive tears of the posterior-superior rotator cuff, in Warner JJP, Iannotti JP, Gerber C (eds): *Complex and Revision Problems in Shoulder Surgery.* Philadelphia, PA, Lippincott-Raven, 1997, pp 177–202.)

function. This kind of individual is likely to have good quality tendon tissue that will be elastic and easily mobilized and repaired.

DIAGNOSIS: IMPORTANT POINTS AND PITFALLS

Not all of these patients with a massive tear that involves the supraspinatus and infraspinatus will have a painful arc and positive impingement signs.[45] Some of these patients may present with a painless pseudoparalysis (Fig. 37, A-D).

Physical examination may actually be accurate in defining the extent of a rotator cuff tear. It is important to recognize that a painful shoulder may appear to be much weaker than it really is, because pain inhibition will prevent good effort by the patient when muscle strength is assessed.[49] Accurate determination of strength therefore requires an initial impingement test to be performed by injecting 10 to 15cc of 1% xylocaine into the subacromial space 10 minutes before examining a patient's strength and active motion.[1,45] Active motion should be assessed with specific attention to scapulothoracic and trunk substitution patterns in individuals with poor glenohumeral motion resulting from a massive rotator cuff tears. Any differences between passive and active motion arcs are very valuable observations and can give specific information regarding the size and location of the tendon tear.[50] For example, a patient who has greater passive than active external rotation when the arm is positioned in adduction will have a large or massive rotator cuff tear that involves at least the supraspinatus (Fig. 37, D and E). Such a lag sign for external rotation when the shoulder is abducted to 90° in the scapular plane is pathognomonic for a massive tear that extends into the infraspinatus as well (Fig. 37, F and G). This observation has been described as the "horn blower's sign" (signe du clarone).[7,26]

RADIOGRAPHS

Routine radiographs that should be obtained include the supraspinatus outlet view[45,51–54] to clarify acromial morphology as hooked, curved, or flat, and thus give information about the shape of the supraspinatus outlet; the caudal tilt AP view[55] to demonstrate the anterior-inferior projection of the acromion; an AP view of the acromioclavicular joint to determine the presence of concomitant acromioclavicular joint disease and an inferior osteophyte that may be contributing to outlet impingement; an axillary view to demonstrate the presence of an os acromiale, which can be present in up to 19% of patients with a large rotator cuff tear;[56–58] and a true AP view of the shoulder. This last radiograph is obtained as the patient attempts to abduct the shoulder, and it can give useful biomechanical information about glenohumeral motion. Superior humeral head displacement will be diagnostic of at least a supraspinatus tear. The AHI may be reproducibly measured when the shoulder is in neutral rotation and adducted at the side, and this measurement may be correlated with the size of a rotator cuff tear (Fig. 38). For example, a normal AHI is ≥ 7 mm, but one that is observed to be less than 3 mm is always associated with a massive tear involving the infraspinatus, and such superior subluxation is static[31] (Fig. 34, B).

LeClerq[16] described an abduction view obtained with the patient's arm at 30° of abduction and holding a 2 kg weight in the hand. I (JPW) have found a true AP plain radiograph obtained with the arm actively abducted at least 30° to be a more reproducible measure of superior translation of the humeral head. The center of the humeral head can be consistently measured relative to the center of the glenoid, and concerns about the obliquity of the x-ray film are not a problem as may be the case when measuring the AHI.[15–18]

ARTHROGRAM AND MAGNETIC RESONANCE IMAGING

Although the arthrogram is very sensitive and cost-effective for detection of full-thickness rotator cuff tears, it is invasive, it can miss pathology of the subscapularis tendon, and it does not predict the size of the tendon tear.[59]

MRI is sensitive, specific, and accurate;[59] however, it is expensive, and its usefulness is very dependent on the skill and experience of the radiologist as well as the power of the magnet.

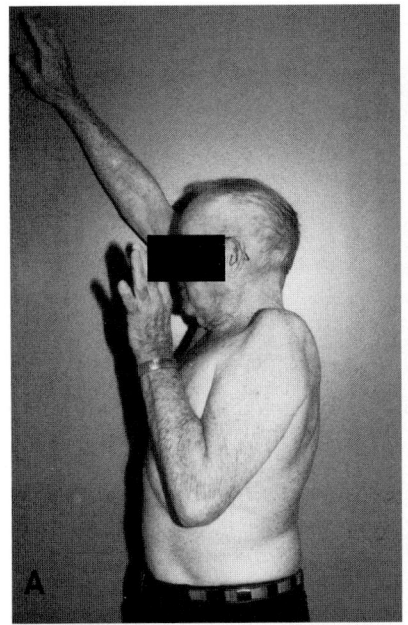
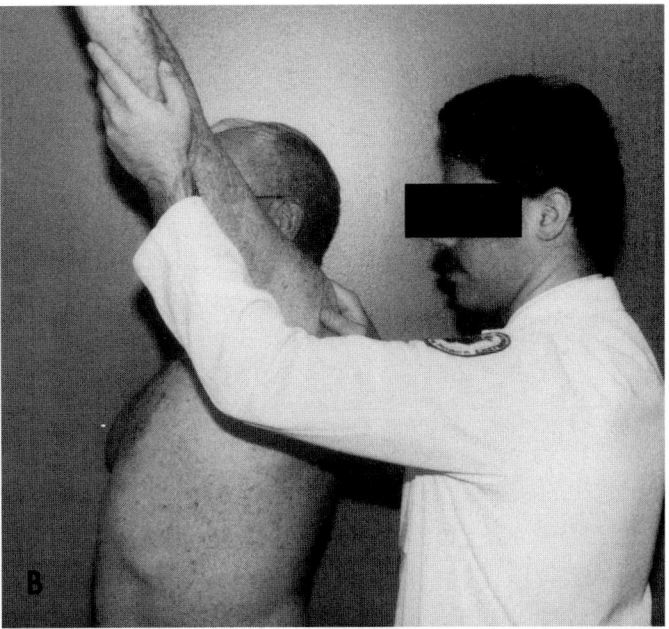
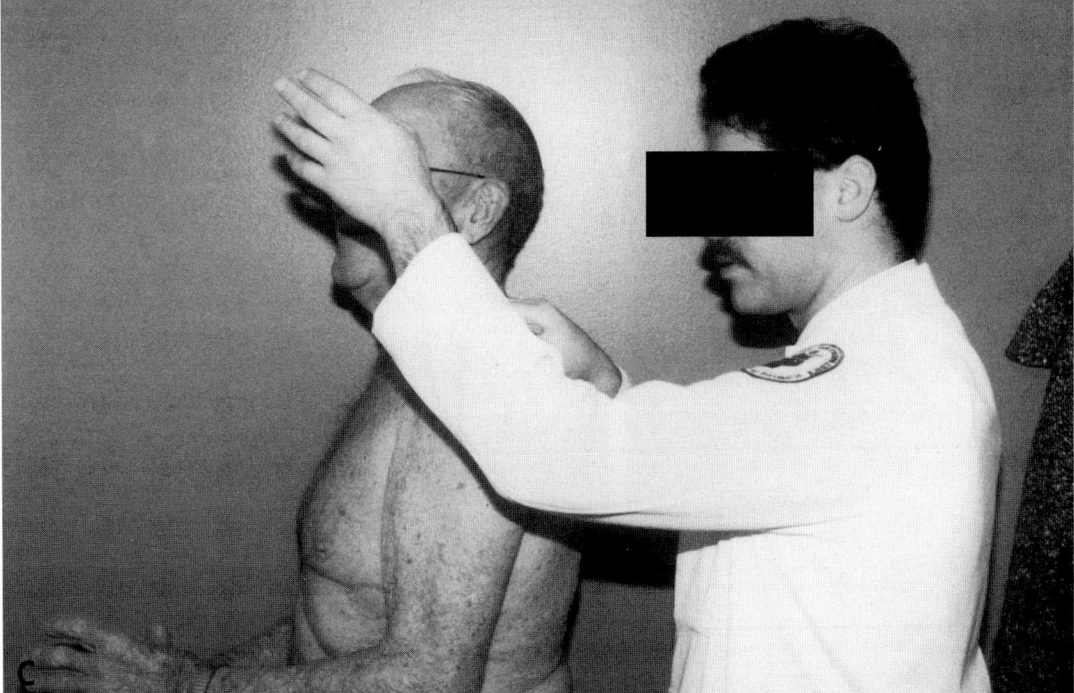

FIGURE 37
68-year-old man with a chronic massive left rotator cuff tear that involves the supraspinatus and infraspinatus. He has poor active motion and minimal pain (**A** and **B**). Passive flexion is preserved (**C**); however, he cannot maintain this position against gravity.

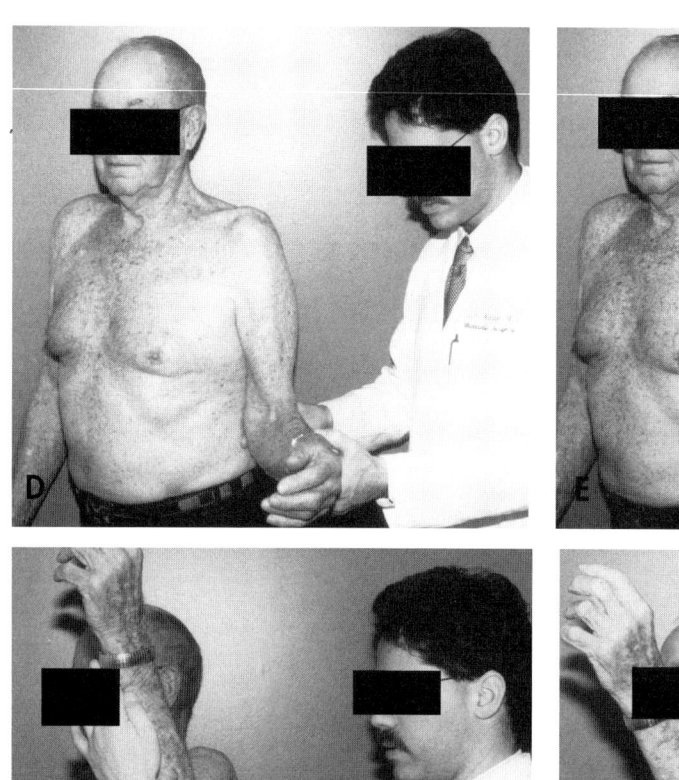
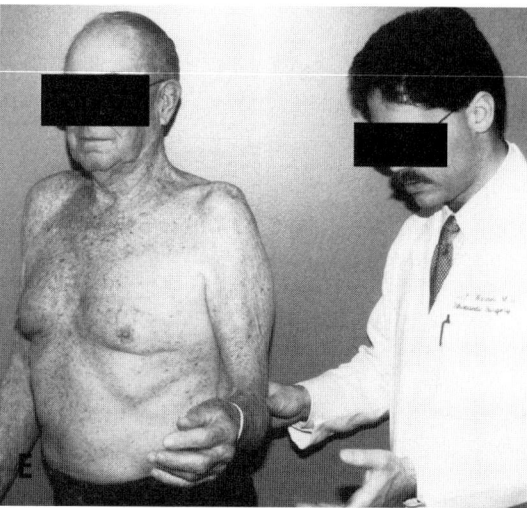
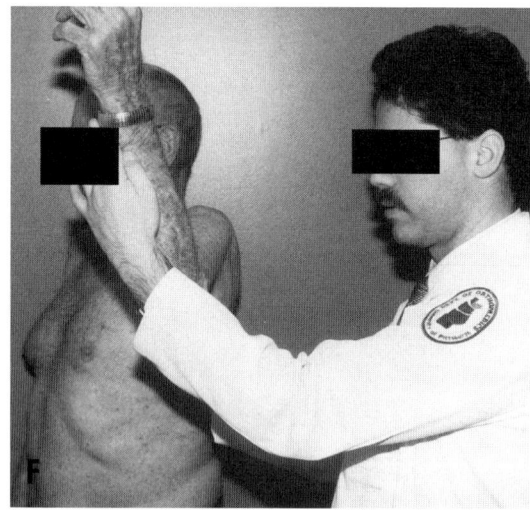
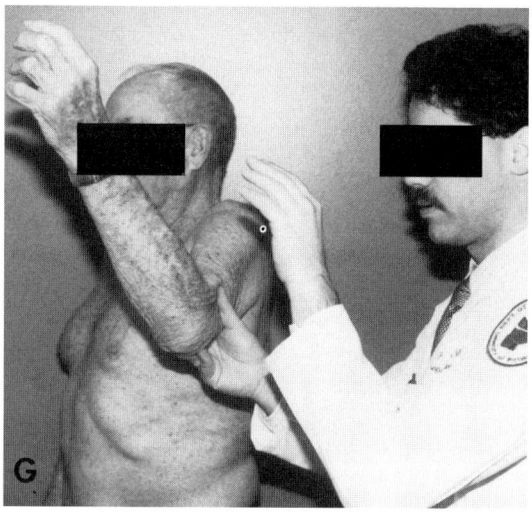

FIGURE 37 (CONTINUED)
He has a 30° lag between passive and active external rotation with the arm at the side.(**D** and **E**); and also a 30° lag between passive and active external rotation with the shoulder in abduction (**F** and **G**).

MRI may be particularly useful in confirmation of the size of the rotator cuff tear and in defining the degree of muscle atrophy and fatty degeneration in patients suspected to have a massive rotator cuff tear.[17,41,60] This latter observation may have direct impact on the nature of subsequent surgical treatment, and the images that appear to give the most information about muscle are those made in the oblique, sagittal plane (Fig. 34).

SURGICAL CONSIDERATIONS

PATIENT POSITIONING

The patient is positioned on a long bean bag in an upright seated position on a bed, with the head of the bed at about a 45° angle. The bean bag is then molded so that the front and back of the shoulder are free and the head is supported. Passive range of motion is first assessed under

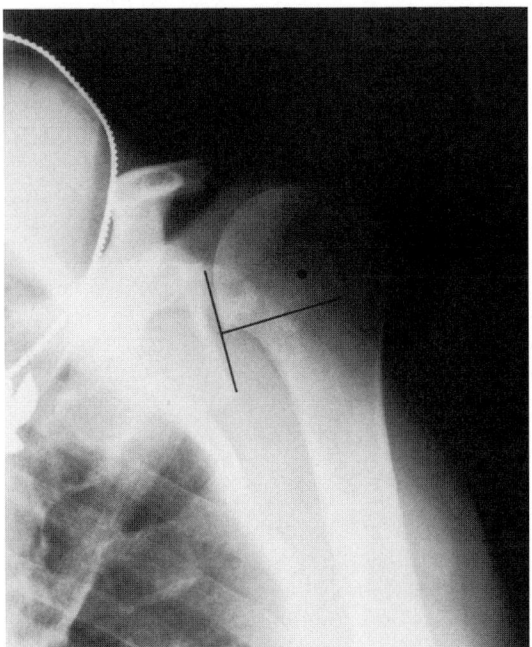

FIGURE 38
True anteroposterior radiograph with the shoulder abducted in a patient with a chronic massive posterior-superior rotator cuff tear. There is superior movement of the center of the humeral head relative to the equator of the glenoid.

anesthesia, and if there is any loss of passive motion the shoulder is manipulated before an incision is made. In some cases, especially after prior surgery, a formal release of adhesions is required during the surgery.

SURGICAL APPROACH

The skin incision is in an anterior oblique orientation in Langer's lines, and it begins over the top of the acromion and continues to just lateral to the coracoid process (Fig. 39). Incisions that cross laterally over the top of the shoulder are generally avoided because these are nonextensile if a combined anterior approach is required for surgical repair of a subscapularis tear. Furthermore, this kind of incision often causes a thick, noncosmetic scar.[61,62] Subcutaneous flaps are mobilized over the acromioclavicular joint and laterally over the palpable lateral extent of the acromion. This is an important step, especially in revision cases where an injured and retracted deltoid muscle

may be adherent to the overlying skin. The deltoid is elevated off the top of the acromion using an electrocautery device, beginning just lateral to the acromioclavicular joint and about 5 mm posterior to the anterior edge. This step allows a thick cuff of tissue to be elevated for subsequent transosseous repair at the completion of the procedure (Fig. 39). Alternatively, if the coracoacromial ligament is to be preserved in cases where it may be an important restraint to superior translation, the deltoid is split in line with its fibers beginning at the lateral edge of the acromion. The anterior deltoid is left attached and undisturbed in this case.

The standard approach of deltoid detachment involves raising a subperiosteal flap off the acromion and splitting the deltoid laterally for a distance of 2 to 3 cm. Extension of the deltoid split further than 5 cm endangers the axillary nerve. It is particularly helpful to split the deltoid laterally and remove the anterior deltoid as a sleeve off the acromion, because this procedure allows much better access to the posterior region of the rotator cuff than that permitted by a more anterior split of the deltoid (Fig. 39). The coracoacromial ligament will come off with the deltoid detachment, and it can then be resected or repaired along with the deltoid at the end of the procedure. In cases of complete rotator cuff loss with superior migration of the humeral head, this ligament should not be removed because it functions as the last barrier to unchecked anterior-superior translation of the humeral head[1,27] (Fig. 35).

A periosteal elevator is then placed underneath the acromion to strip any adhesions between it and the rotator cuff. This step is important to avoid inadvertent injury to the rotator cuff, which may be scarred to the undersurface of the acromion. In patients with significant acromioclavicular joint pain and arthritis, the periosteal incision is extended from the acromion over the distal clavicle, periosteal-fascial flaps of deltoid and trapezius are elevated, and the distal 10 to 15 mm of clavicle is excised. Sharp dissection is then used to mobilize the subdeltoid interval because adhesions can connect the deltoid to

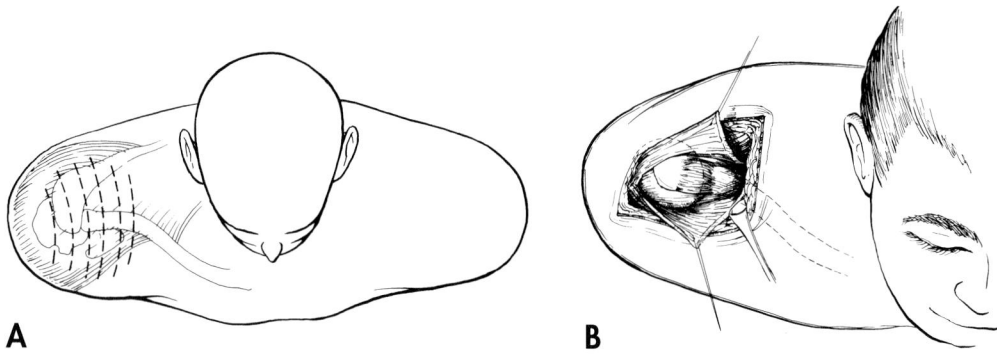

FIGURE 39

A, Incision in Langer's lines for best cosmesis. **B,** Deltoid mobilization through subperiosteal elevation with split directly through the lateral deltoid. (Reproduced with permission from Warner JJP, Gerber C: Massive tears of the posterior-superior rotator cuff, in Warner JJP, Iannotti JP, Gerber C (eds): *Complex and Revision Problems in Shoulder Surgery*. Philadelphia, PA, Lippincott-Raven, 1997, pp 177–202.)

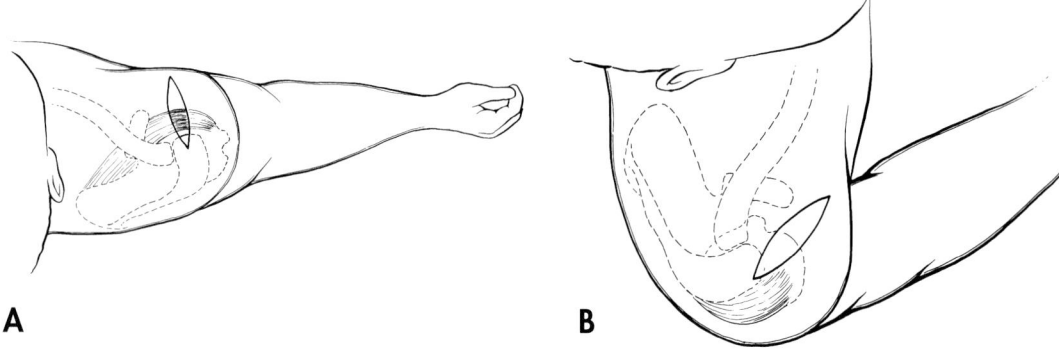

FIGURE 40

External rotation of the arm **(A)** allows visualization of the subscapularis, whereas internal rotation **(B)** allows visualization of the infraspinatus. (Reproduced with permission from Warner JJP, Gerber C: Massive tears of the posterior-superior rotator cuff, in Warner JJP, Iannotti JP, Gerber C (eds): *Complex and Revision Problems in Shoulder Surgery*. Philadelphia, PA, Lippincott-Raven, 1997, pp 177–202.)

the proximal humerus. In some individuals with passive loss of motion, especially in revision cases, these two steps can partially improve motion. A flexible retractor is then placed underneath the acromion, and an acromioplasty is performed. The amount of acromial resection should be individualized. An oscillating saw allows this step to be precise, and the acromioplasty is performed to create a flat undersurface. The thick-ness of the remaining acromion is assessed, and at the completion of the rotator cuff tear repair, the clearance of the tendon underneath the acromion is assessed by rotating the arm. Further bone removal is performed as necessary.

In many cases the bursa may be quite hyper-trophic and thick. It is carefully defined from the underlying rotator cuff and then excised. The rotator cuff tear configuration and quality of the tendon tissue can then be defined by placing several sutures into the tendon tissue and rotating the arm to visualize the extent of the tear (Fig. 40). The important characteristics of the tear are its actual size once debridement of the irregular edges is performed, the number of tendons involved, and the quality of the tendon tissue. These observations define the reparability of the tear. Degree of tendon retraction and tear size are actually less important than tissue quality. For example, some "massive tears" (> 5 cm diameter) can be repaired easily because once they are mobilized through formal tendon release, the tendons are thick, robust, and elastic. Conversely, some medium (2 to 3 cm) and large tears (3 to 5 cm) can be difficult to securely repair because of poor tendon tissue that is thin, friable, and inelastic even after extensive intra- and extra-articular releases.

The techniques of mobilization and release of a chronically retracted rotator cuff tear have been well described by Neer and associates.[1,63] The coracohumeral ligament is divided first by pulling on the sutures that have been placed in the supraspinatus tendon and cutting soft-tissue extensions to the base of the coracoid process[63] (Fig. 41, A). If sufficient tendon length is not obtained to allow reinsertion into the greater tuberosity, the interval between the superior labrum and rotator cuff is divided sharply (Fig. 41, B). Care should be taken not to injure the long head of the biceps tendon. A periosteal elevator is then placed into this interval and pushed medially to elevate the supraspinatus off the lateral supraspinatus fossa (Fig. 41, C and D). When performing this maneuver it is important not to advance the instruments more than 2 cm laterally, because there is a risk of injury to the suprascapular nerve[64] (Fig. 41, E). If mobilization of the supraspinatus tendon is still insufficient for its repair, an "interval slide" can be performed by dividing tissue in the rotator interval (interval between subscapularis and supraspinatus)[2] (Fig. 41, F and G). Similar steps can be performed for mobilization of the infraspinatus.

In cases where visualization of the retracted tendon is difficult, resection of the acromioclavic-

ular joint permits direct observation of the superior glenoid and lateral aspect of the supraspinatus fossa. The supraspinatus tendon can then be mobilized directly into its fossa. A specially designed retractor (Subacromial spreader, Protek Company, Switzerland) that allows the humeral head to be distracted inferiorly away from the acromion can greatly improve the surgeon's view (Fig. 42). Alternatively, a laminar spreader can be used with the limbs placed on the acromion and the greater tuberosity.

In cases where the tendon tissue remains insufficient for an adequate repair, some surgeons[31] have suggested mobilizing the entire muscle belly of the supraspinatus and infraspinatus out of their respective fossae so that they can be moved laterally. I (JPW) never perform this maneuver because there may be a real risk to the suprascapular neurovascular pedicle. Furthermore, lateral transposition of the entire muscle tendon unit will shorten its lever arm and result in severe weakness.

TECHNICAL ASPECTS OF THE TENDON REPAIR TO BONE

Following formal releases, the cuff tissue should be mobilized sufficiently so that it can reach the greater tuberosity with the patient's arm at the side. Repair is then performed to bone. The ideal repair, as defined by Gerber and associates,[65] should satisfy three important criteria: (1) it should have high initial fixation strength; (2) it should allow minimal gap formation at the bone-suture-tendon interface; and (3) it should maintain mechanical stability until healing of the tendon to bone is complete. Recent observations have suggested that tendon repair to bone may fail more often than suspected.[4,66] Failure can occur at one of three points in the repair: (1) the suture or knot may fail; (2) the tendon may fail, allowing the sutures to pull through it; or (3) the bone may fail, allowing the suture to pull through it. These weak links in the repair have been defined and quantified in several in vitro studies.[65,67–69] Methods to maximize repair strength at each point are described in the following text.

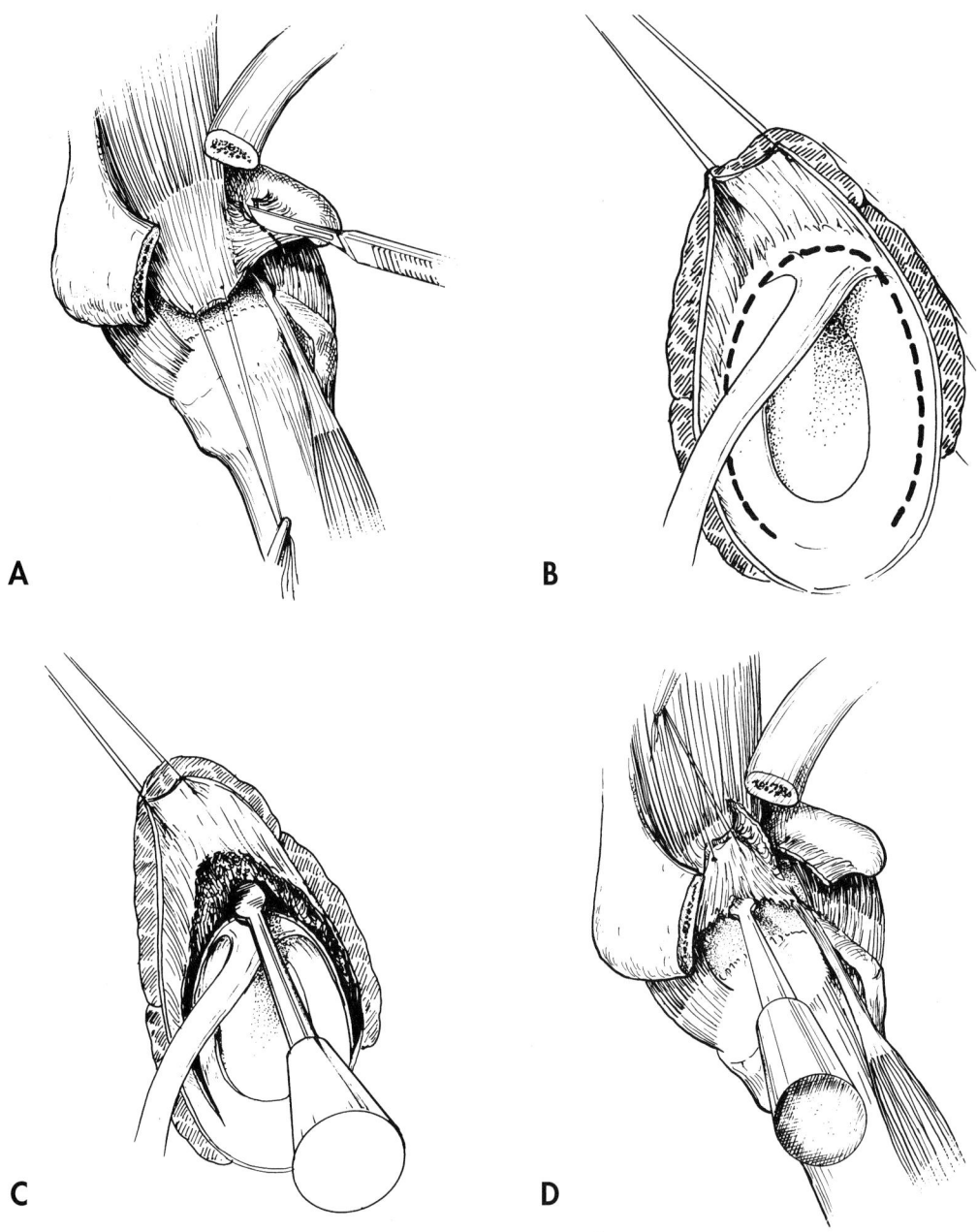

FIGURE 41

Mobilization of a chronic retracted rotator cuff tendon tear. **A,** Sutures are placed in the end of the supraspinatus and tension is applied to the tendon to demonstrate the coracohumeral ligament under tension. This ligament is then divided. Acromial and clavicle resections are exagerated to show the surgical technique in this drawing. **B,** Intra-articular release of the tendon is performed by sharp incision between the labrum and the rotator cuff. **C** and **D,** An elevator is then placed into the supraspinatus fossa to mobilize the tendon. (Reproduced with permission from Warner JJP, Gerber C: Massive tears of the posterior-superior rotator cuff, in Warner JJP, Iannotti JP, Gerber C (eds): *Complex and Revision Problems in Shoulder Surgery.* Philadelphia, PA, Lippincott-Raven, 1997, pp 177–202.)

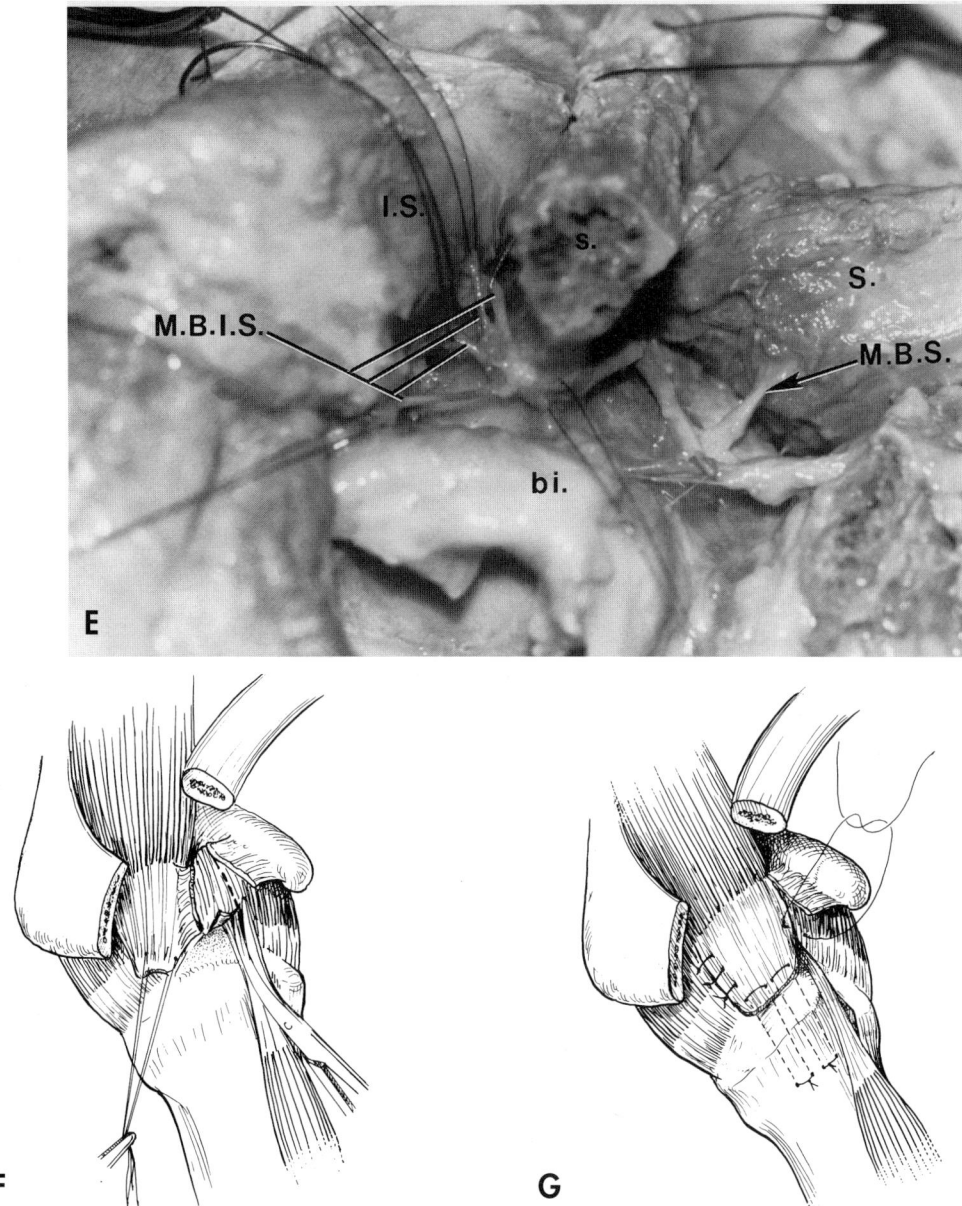

FIGURE 41 (CONTINUED)

Mobilization of a chronic retracted rotator cuff tendon tear. **E,** The suprscapular motor branches to the infraspinatus (MBIS) are in close proximity to the superior glenoid and biceps origin (bi). The acromion has been removed in this cadaver shoulder and the infraspinatus (IS) and supraspinatus (S) tendons have been detached from their insertions. The motor branch to the supraspinatus (MBS) is also shown. **F,** Additional mobilization can be obtained by dividing the rotator interval. **G,** Tendon repair is then performed to bone as well as by side to side tendon sutures. (Figure 41E is reproduced with permission from Warner JJP, Krushell RJ, Masquelet A, Gerber C: Anatomy and relationships of the suprascapular nerve: Anatomical constraints to mobiliization of the supraspinatus and infraspinatus muscles in the management of massive rotator cuff tears. *J Bone Joint Surg* 1992;74A:36–45. Figures 41F–G are reproduced with permission from Warner JJP, Gerber C: Massive tears of the posterior-superior rotator cuff, in Warner JJP, Iannotti JP, Gerber C (eds): *Complex and Revision Problems in Shoulder Surgery.* Philadelphia, PA, Lippincott-Raven, 1997, pp 177–202.)

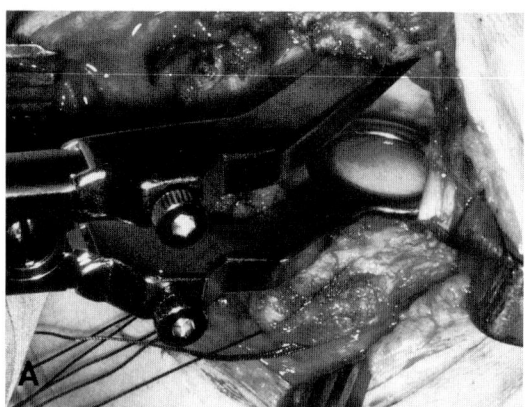
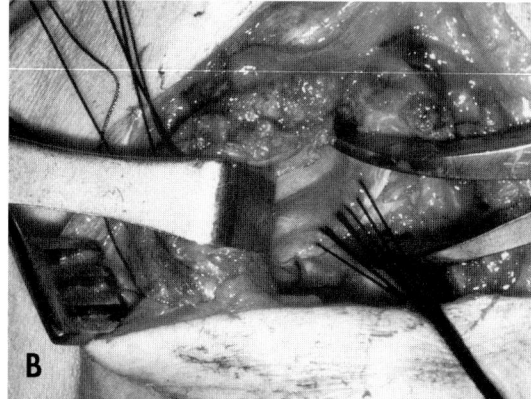

FIGURE 42
A, Retracted massive rotator cuff tear in a right shoulder. The subacromial distraction device is in place with the ring-shaped limb on the humeral head and the spiked limb underneath the acromion. **B,** After tendon releases and mobilization the edge of the tendon can be seen. The position of the subacromial distraction device has been changed.

Suture

Sutures smaller than #1 or #2 do not provide sufficient strength for repair of large retracted tears. Monofilament absorbable suture materials lose 50% of their in vitro ultimate tensile strength at 3 to 4 weeks after implantation.[70,71] Although some surgeons[17] believe this time course is acceptable for use in rotator cuff tear repair, Gerber and associates[65] have shown that the extensibility or plastic deformation of this suture material permits large gap formation of the repair when it is subject to cyclical loading. Therefore, these suture materials should not be used for repair of large retracted tears. Braided, nonabsorbable polyester of #3 or #2 size has the best combined ultimate tensile strength and stiffness.

Tendon Suture Techniques

Most suturing techniques used for repair of rotator cuff tears are either weak or tend to strangulate the tendon tissue.[65] The optimal suture knot technique is the modified Mason-Allen stitch[65] (Fig. 43) because it results in twice the holding power of a simple stitch. Furthermore, because it grasps few fiber bundles it should cause less strangulation of the tissue than other grasping sutures.[72]

Transosseous Repair

When there is a long-standing massive rotator cuff tear, the bone of the proximal humerus may be quite osteoporotic as a result of lack of loading from loss of tendon attachment and reduced use of the arm. In this situation the holding power of the bony cortex and cancellous tuberosity is poor. Poor holding power especially may be a problem if one of the popular suture anchor systems is used. In these cases, contrary to the situation in an individual with an acute rotator cuff tear and thicker tuberosity bone, bone fixation may fail at loads half that of standard transosseous cortical fixation repairs[65] (Fig. 44). In a patient with an osteopenic greater tuberosity the transosseous suture configuration can greatly influence the initial strength of the overall repair. If the sutures are passed from the greater tuberosity so that they exit the proximal humerus at least 2 to 3 cm from the tip of the greater tuberosity, and if they are tied over a bone bridge of at least 1 cm, the pull-out strength of transosseous fixation can be increased by a factor of three.[67] This increase is a result of the increasing thickness of the cortex as the surgeon moves distal to the tip of the greater tuberosity (Fig. 45). In cases where there is marked osteopenia, cortical augmentation can further improve the holding strength of sutures. In this situation, a plastic ligament button can be cut into the shape of a rectangle, and the sutures are placed through it so that when they are tied down the button distributes the load over a broader area of the humeral cortex (Fig. 45).

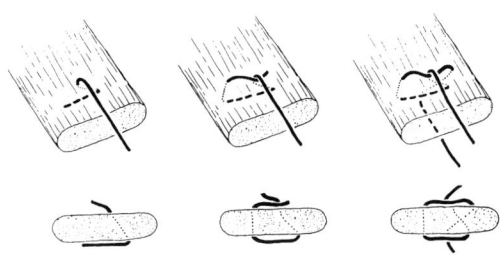

FIGURE 43
Technique of modified Mason-Allen suture. (Reproduced with permission from Gerber C, Schneeberger AG, Beck M, Schlegel U: Mechanical strength of repairs of the rotator cuff. *J Bone Joint Surg* 1994;76B:371–380.)

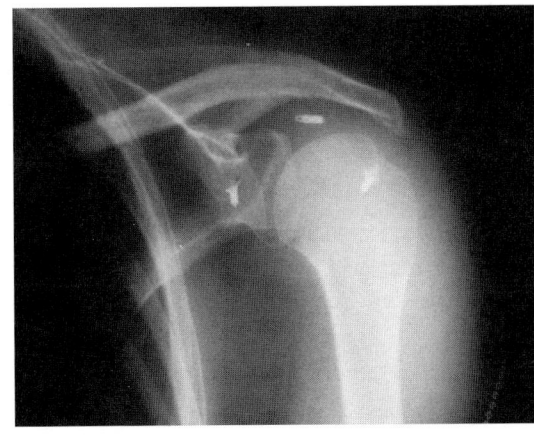

FIGURE 44
Loose bone anchors after rotator cuff repair.

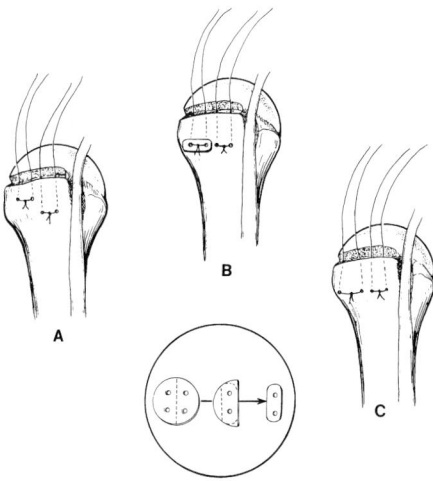

FIGURE 45
A, Distal placement of sutures improves holding power in bone. **B,** A plastic ligament button can be used to augment the cortical strength of a transosseous suture repair (inset). **C,** Bone bridge should be ≥ 1 cm in diameter. (Reproduced with permission from Warner JJP, Gerber C: Massive tears of the posterior-superior rotator cuff, in Warner JJP, Iannotti JP, Gerber C: *Complex and Revision Problems in Shoulder Surgery.* Philadelphia, PA, Lippincott-Raven, 1997, pp 177–202.)

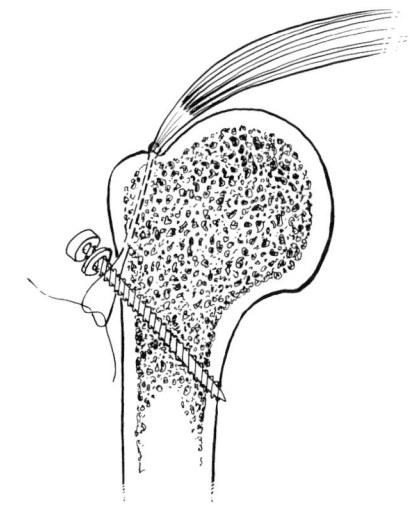

FIGURE 46
Salvage of transosseous repair in case of poor greater tuberosity bone. A bicortical screw and washer are used. The threads on the screw should be limited to the distal half of the screw in order to avoid cutting the suture. (Reproduced with permission from Warner JJP, Gerber C: Massive tears of the posterior-superior rotator cuff, in Warner JJP, Iannotti JP, Gerber C (eds): *Complex and Revision Problems in Shoulder Surgery.* Philadelphia, PA, Lippincott-Raven, 1997, pp 177–202.)

This augmentation can improve pull-out strength by a factor of two.[65,67,69] In rare cases where there is severe bone loss from prior surgery, it may be impossible to tie sutures over a cortical bone bridge. In this situation a helpful revision technique is to place a bicortical screw and washer into the proximal humerus and then pull the sutures through the bony trough and tie them around the screw and washer post (Fig. 46).

CONFIGURATION OF THE REPAIR

In a massive rotator cuff tear, the tendons pull away from their insertion not only in a lateral to medial direction but also in an anterior to posterior direction. The resulting massive tear configuration occurs because of a boutonniere-type effect. This is why meticulous release of the supraspinatus and infraspinatus may allow closure of massive tears. In many cases, these tendons retract anteriorly and posteriorly, respectively, and once mobilized they can be brought over the top of the humerus and closed in a side-to-side fashion from the medial apex of the tear in a lateral direction. This procedure will then leave a cuff of tissue that can be inserted, without tension, directly into the greater tuberosity (Fig. 47).

The torn edges of the tendon may also become delaminated, so care should be taken to define the tendon tear in the plane of the tendon and to capture the entire thickness of the tendon with each stitch. Our preference is to group sutures into pairs with two sets for each tendon. Thus, in a massive tear involving two tendons, two sets of two sutures (total of four) each are placed in the supraspinatus and infraspinatus tendons. Instead of creating a deep trough in the greater tuberosity, the residual soft tissue of the tendon tear is removed and the bone of the greater tuberosity is abraded just medial to the original anatomic insertion of the tendon. This abrasion promotes soft-tissue to bone healing but does not remove the structural integrity of the cortical bone of the greater tuberosity. A deep trough risks fracture of the tuberosity and also requires further advancement of the tendon into the trough for good bone contact. For suture passage, I (JPW) prefer a special suture passer (Concept Rotator Cuff Repair System; Linvatec Corp, Largo, FL) that allows the sutures to be placed so that they exit the lateral humeral cortex at least 2 cm distal to the greater tuberosity. The sutures are kept in pairs and passed into the greater tuberosity and out the lateral cortex of the humerus, and no more than four holes are made in the humerus (Fig. 45). This procedure allows for a cortical bone bridge of at least 1 cm between each set of sutures.

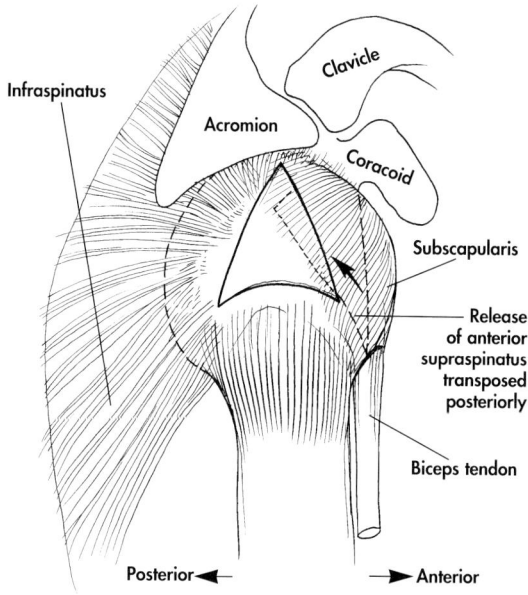

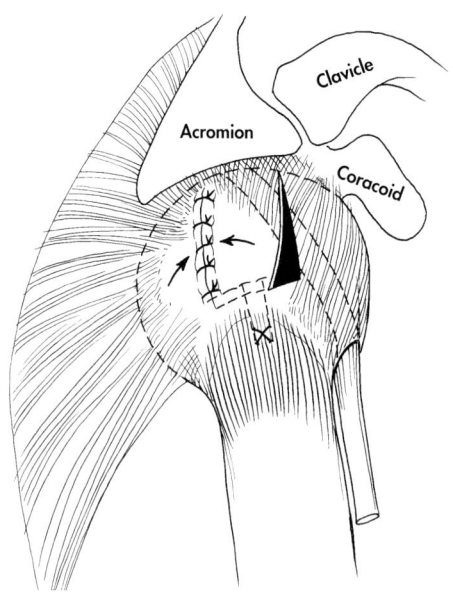

FIGURE 47

Closure of the rotator cuff in an anterior-posterior direction as well as medial to lateral direction.

The sutures are tied down while maintaining the shoulder in abduction. The arm then is brought down to the side and moved through a passive arc of motion to determine where the repair comes under tension. This information is used to guide postoperative passive motion therapy by the physical therapist.

DELTOID CLOSURE

Because deltoid closure is the final and critical step to any rotator cuff repair, it should be performed in a manner that results in a secure and strong repair.[73] I (JPW) prefer to place two to four transosseous #2 or #3, nonabsorbable, braided sutures through the acromion and then fix the deltoid back with Mason-Allen stitches (Fig. 48). The lateral deltoid split is then reapproximated and, if an acromioclavicular joint resection has been performed, the trapezius and deltoid fascia are closed in pants-over-vest fashion using nonabsorbable suture.

POSTOPERATIVE TREATMENT

The use of an abduction pillow following repair of a massive rotator cuff tear remains a point of controversy. Some surgeons believe it is contraindicated, because they assume it is being used to protect a tendon repair that would be under tension if the shoulder is adducted. As previously described, the criteria for a tendon to be reparable are that it can be sufficiently mobilized so that it can be repaired without tension when the arm is at the patient's side. The abduction pillow then is used for several reasons. First, it places the muscle-tendon units at a lax position (unstretched), which probably reduces the likelihood of reflexive muscle contraction during the postoperative course. Second, it may promote increased blood flow to the tendon repair because there will be reduced tension on the repair. For these reasons, I (JPW) prefer to use an abduction pillow for the first 6 weeks following repair of a massive, chronic tendon tear.

Passive motion is begun on the first postoperative day and is continued for 6 weeks. In such cases of a massive tear, pendulums, pulleys, and self-assisted range of motion exercises are not permitted because some degree of active muscle contraction is likely to occur and this contraction may risk the integrity of the repaired tendon. The limits of this passive motion are clearly defined for the therapist, based on our intraoperative observations after repair. No attempt is made to aggressively stretch the shoulder beyond these limits during the initial 6-week postoperative period. After 6 weeks, the patient begins to use the arm

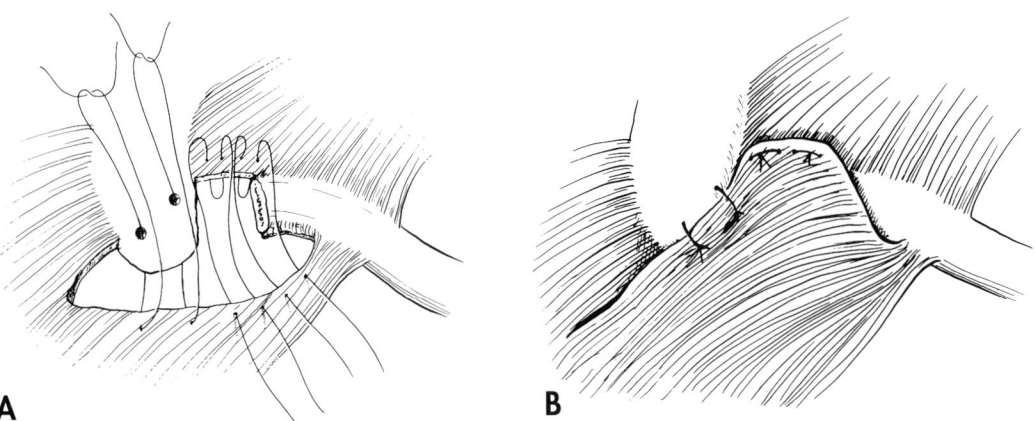

A   **B**

FIGURE 48

A, Transosseous repair of the deltoid to the acromion and closure of the defect of the distal clavicle. **B,** Deltoid is brought into the acromioclavicular joint defect. (Reproduced with permission from Warner JJP, Gerber C: Massive tears of the posterior-superior rotator cuff, in Warner JJP, Iannotti JP, Gerber C (eds): *Complex and Revision Problems in Shoulder Surgery.* Philadelphia, PA, Lippincott-Raven, 1997, pp 177–202.)

for activities of daily living and performs active-assisted motion exercises. Strengthening is delayed until 3 months after surgery, and then it begins with elastic bands only. Free weights are avoided for at least 4 to 6 months after surgery. A common cause of failure in the initial 6 months after surgery is excessive overloading by use of free weights. Patients who want to are permitted to swim or play racquet sports at 8 months after their surgery. In general, strength gains can continue to be significant for over 1 year after the surgery.

CLINICAL OUTCOME AFTER REPAIR

Recently, the experience in both Europe (M Mansat, MD, unpublished data, 1992) and the United States (FA Matsen III, MD, unpublished data, 1992) has been presented. Multicenter analyses were performed to determine results after surgical repair of combined tears of the supraspinatus and infraspinatus in patients who also had biceps tendon disease. In Europe, the treatment of 218 cases in eight different centers consisted of direct tendon repair or local tendon transfer in 63% of cases, deltoid flap reconstruction of the rotator cuff in 13%, Debyre muscle slide in 8%, debridement in 16%, and free tendon graft in 1%. Most of these patients had range of motion greater than 120° of flexion, although most had marked abduction weakness. In the United States, 61 cases from four centers were treated only with direct tendon repair or local tendon transfer. Ultrasound was performed at 5 years after surgery and demonstrated that the tendon repair was intact in only 50% of those patients who had an isolated supraspinatus tear. The repair was intact in only 15% of those with both the supraspinatus and infraspinatus tendons torn. An intact tendon repair correlated with better function.

TREATMENT OF IRREPARABLE TEARS

SURGICAL TECHNIQUES

The term "irreparable" rotator cuff tears is not synonymous with "massive" rotator cuff tears.

Intraoperative factors that determine a rotator cuff tear's reparability are tendon tissue quality and retraction and surgeon's skill.[7] In fact, the reparability of a tendon tear can be predicted preoperatively with relatively good accuracy. In general, preoperative factors that predict that a tendon tear will be massive and "irreparable" are radiographic demonstration of static superior subluxation with an acromiohumeral interval of < 3 mm, profound loss of external rotation strength, and MRI evidence of extreme muscle fatty degeneration and atrophy (Fig. 34). These factors predict that the tendon tissue will be of poor quality. Furthermore, if there is moderate or nearly complete replacement of a muscle by fat, it is unlikely that it can actively function even if its tendon is repaired. Thus, even if torn tendon tissue can be reapproximated by aggressive surgical mobilization, these tears are likely to be "functionally irreparable". In fact, Goutallier and associates[41] have shown that this chronic muscle degeneration does not recover following surgical repairs. Overall, about 5% of all rotator cuff are either structurally or functionally irreparable.

Treatment of these patients must be individualized because the degree of disability and pain may vary. Some of these individuals will have poor function but minimal pain, and in these cases we would recommend against any surgery (Fig. 34). A few will have good function and minimal pain, and they also should not have any surgical treatment (Fig. 35, A). Those patients who have both pain and poor function in association with arthritis may be best managed by hemiarthroplasty replacement using a large modular head and preserving the coracoacromial ligament as a fulcrum for rotation of the prosthetic humeral head.[27]

In patients with painful and dysfunctional shoulders and tendon tears that cannot be closed by standard methods, several types of local tendon transfers have been recommended. These have included a superior transposition of the upper two thirds of the subscapularis[30,36,74] in cases where the supraspinatus cannot be repaired (Fig. 49) and superior transposition of the teres minor in cases where the infraspinatus cannot be

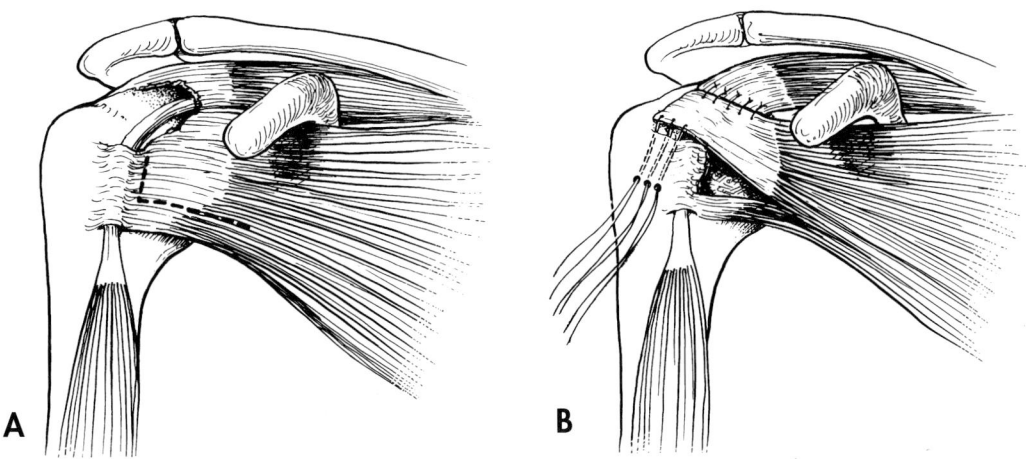

FIGURE 49
Massive supraspinatus tear (**A**) closed with transposition of the upper two thirds of the subscapularis tendon (**B**). (Reproduced with permission from Warner JJP, Gerber C: Massive tears of the posterior-superior rotator cuff, in Warner JJP, Iannotti JP, Gerber C (eds): *Complex and Revision Problems in Shoulder Surgery*. Philadelphia, PA, Lippincott-Raven, 1997, pp 177–202.)

repaired.[36] Although the experience of some surgeons with these transfers has been favorable, I (JPW) believe that such tendon transposition should be avoided because it will weaken the anterior-posterior force couple of the rotator cuff. This couple is very important for stability of the humeral head on the glenoid during abduction.[25] For example, if the infraspinatus is torn, then the teres minor is the only remaining external rotator. Transfer of this tendon unit in a cranial direction in order to close a cuff defect will probably weaken its external rotation function and may even compromise function.

In patients with pain, poor function, prior infection and/or bone loss, and soft-tissue loss from prior surgery, a fusion is an option for treatment if the other shoulder is normal. Such individuals also often have a deltoid injury from prior surgical repair attempts.

Some elderly patients predominantly have pain, and after xylocaine subacromial injection, may have good pain relief and adequate function. An abduction AP plain radiograph will show that the humeral head remains centered on the glenoid because of adequate preservation of the rotator cuff: deltoid force couple. Although these individuals will have large to massive rotator cuff

tears that are potentially reparable, they may prefer not to subject themselves to the surgical morbidity of a massive rotator cuff tear reconstruction. In these select cases, arthroscopic debridement may be a less morbid technique to relieve pain and improve function.[22–24,75] Although strength will not improve, function usually does improve as a result of the removal of the pain and inhibition from mechanical impingement. However, in these patients it is important not to perform too aggressive an acromioplasty and not to excise the coracoacromial ligament, or anterior-superior subluxation of the shoulder may occur. The appropriate patient for this approach is one older than 60 years of age who is less active, with preoperative active flexion of at least 120° (after subacromial xylocaine) and four fifths external rotation strength. Debridement will fail in individuals with very weak external rotation, a positive horn blower's sign, limited active flexion, and radiographic evidence of superior translation of the humeral head (Figs. 33, *B* and 34). Another important point in these individuals is that much of their pain may come from concomitant biceps tendon disease, and either biceps tendon tenotomy or tenodesis may significantly improve their pain.

A select group of individuals will have pain and poor active motion, but good passive motion without any arthritis. These individuals may or may not have had prior surgical attempts that have failed. Physical examination will show marked external rotation weakness and a positive horn blower's sign (Fig. 50), and the MRI will demonstrate severe atrophy and fatty replacement of the supraspinatus and infraspinatus muscles. Some surgeons have recommended tendon grafting techniques in these patients.[35,76–78]

However, it is difficult to understand how this could work when the muscle is no longer functioning normally. We believe that this type of patient may be a good candidate for the latissimus dorsi transfer technique. This extrinsic tendon transfer provides a strong, vascularized tendon that may close the cuff defect as well as act as a humeral head depressor. With an average follow-up of 5 years, Gerber and asssociates[7,26] have shown that results of this procedure are long lasting. The subscapularis tendon and del-

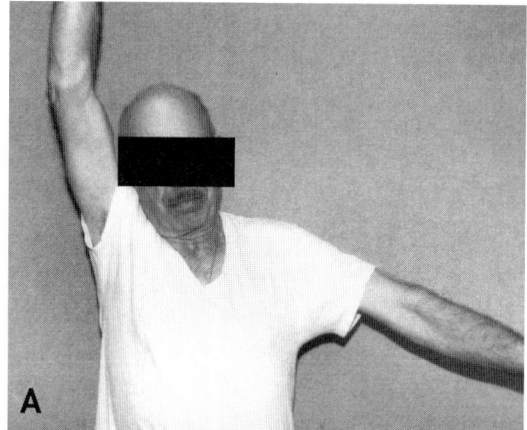
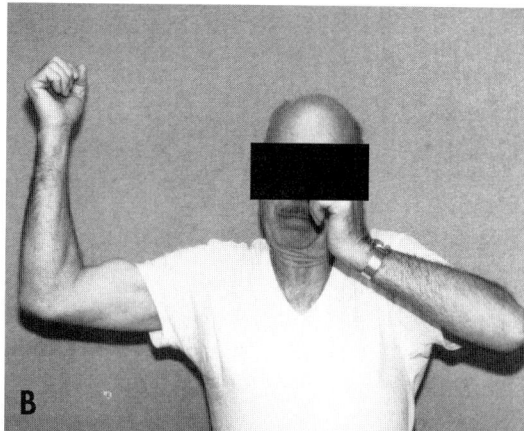
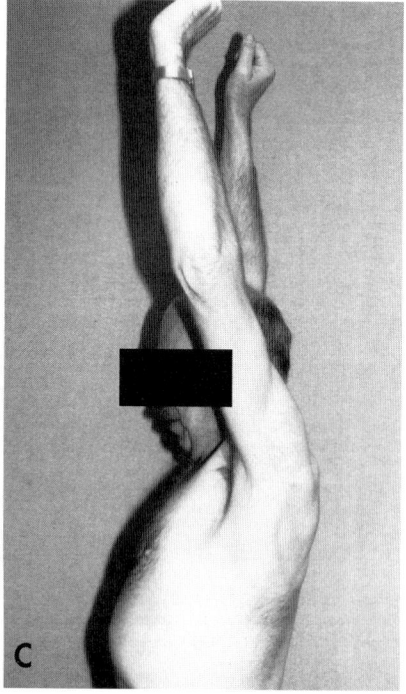
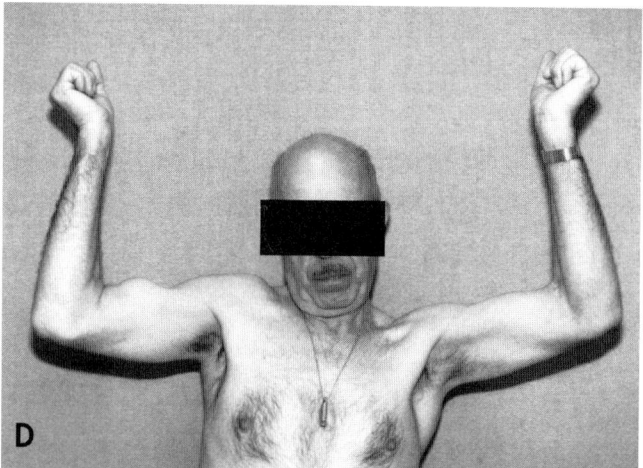

FIGURE 50
68-year-old man with a chronic massive tear of the supraspinatus and infraspinatus tendons of the left shoulder. He has limited abduction (**A**), and a positive "horn blower's sign" (**B**). 3 years after latissimus dorsi transfer he has improved abduction (**C**), and a negative horn blower's sign (**D**).

toid origin must be intact for a patient to be a viable candidate for this tendon transfer.

LATISSIMUS DORSI TENDON TRANSFER

This procedure (Fig. 51) is best performed with the patient in a lateral decubitus position on a long bean bag. A standard anterior-superior approach to the rotator cuff is made as described above, and an attempt is made to mobilize and

repair the tendon tear. The tendon is mobilized as much as possible, and when it is demonstrated that the supraspinatus and infraspinatus cannot be repaired, the decision for latissimus dorsi transfer is made.

The patient's arm is flexed and a posterior L-shaped incision is made over the posterior joint line and along the palpable border of the latissimus dorsi (Fig. 51, *A*). Undermining of the sub-

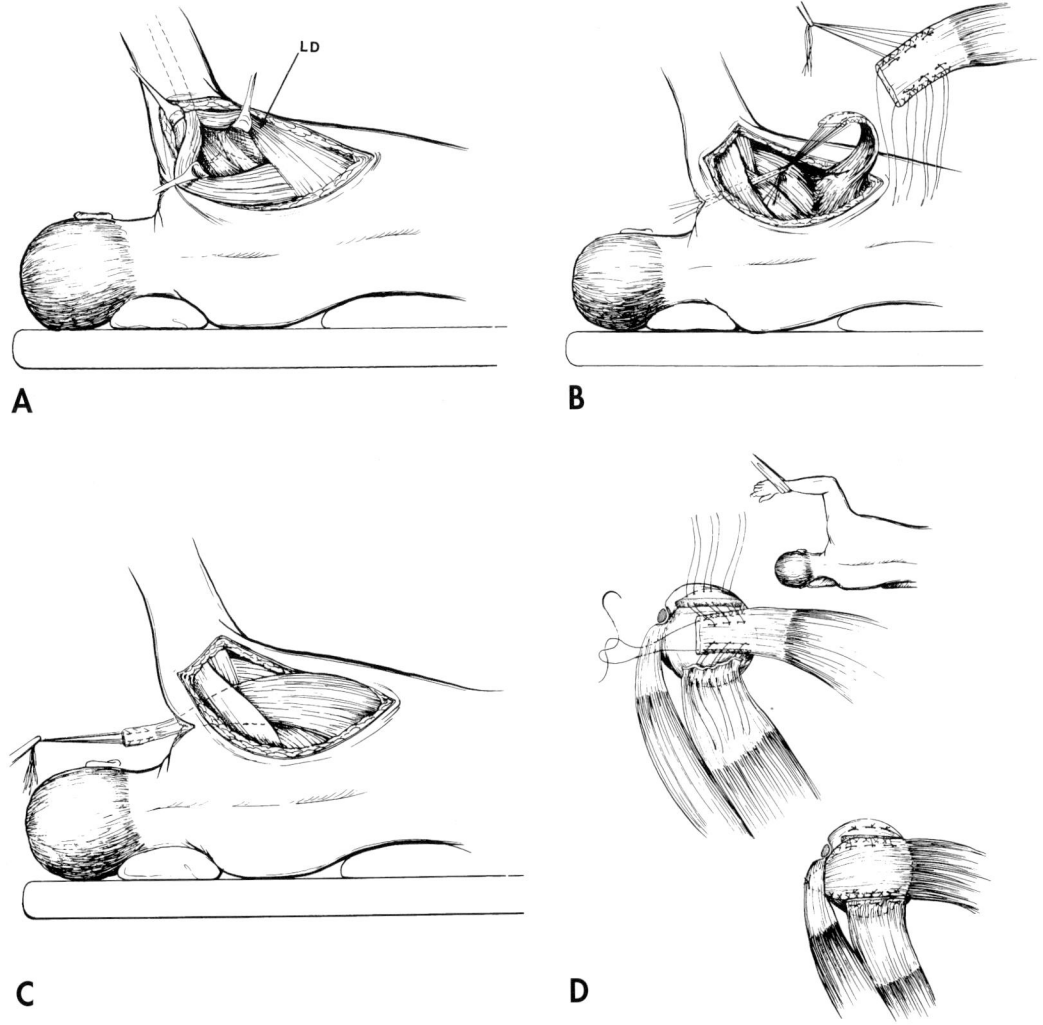

A

B

C

D

FIGURE 51

Technique of latissimus dorsi tendon transfer. **A,** Posterior incision. Latissimus dorsi (LD) is labeled. **B,** Mobilization of the latissimus dorsi tendon and muscle, and placement of sutures (inset). **C,** Transfer of the tendon underneath the deltoid and acromion. **D,** Repair of the latissimus tendon transfer to the greater tuberosity, subscapularis tendon, and residual cuff tissue. (Reproduced with permission from Warner JJP, Gerber C: Massive tears of the posterior-superior rotator cuff, in Warner JJP, Iannotti JP, Gerber C (eds): *Complex and Revision Problems in Shoulder Surgery.* Philadelphia, PA, Lippincott-Raven, 1997, pp 177–202.)

cutaneous layer allows demonstration of the muscles of the posterior deltoid, long head of the triceps, teres minor, teres major, and latissimus dorsi. The latissimus dorsi and teres major muscle bellies are usually closely related to one another, and it is best to identify the plane between the two before dissecting the former. Dissection then proceeds toward the tendon insertion of the latissimus dorsi, and this procedure usually is facilitated by abducting and internally rotating the arm. Long, thin retractors help to visualize the insertion site, and two assistants (one on each side of the table) provide the best retraction. The tendon is detached from the humerus with as much periosteum as possible, and then dissected retrograde to its neurovascular pedicle (Fig. 51, *B*). All attachments to adjacent skin and muscles are released so that the tendon has sufficient excursion for transfer. Generally, the tendon should be mobilized so that it can reach to the level of the posterior acromion to allow for sufficient excursion for its transfer. The tendon is typically long and thin, and its fibers tend to separate from one another if pulled perpendicular to the tendon length. Thus, running sutures of nonabsorbable braided material are placed along each edge of the tendon in order to keep it from splaying apart. Additional sutures are then placed along the lateral edge of the tendon in a Mason-Allen configuration before its passage underneath the acromion (Fig. 51, *B*) because it may be difficult to gain access to the tendon to place sutures in it once it is transferred over the humeral head. A large curved clamp is then passed from the front of the shoulder underneath the acromion and deltoid. The clamp is opened in order to dilate a soft-tissue passage for the tendon. The sutures in the end of the tendon are grasped in the clamp and the tendon is pulled underneath the deltoid and acromion (Fig. 51, *C*). The greater tuberosity is then prepared for the repair as previously described, and the latissimus tendon is sutured into the greater tuberosity using the transosseous method also described earlier (Fig. 51, *D*). The anterior edge of the latissimus tendon is sutured directly into the subscapularis tendon. The arm is maintained in a position of about 60° scapular plane abduction and

45° external rotation. Once the tendon is repaired, any retracted cuff tissue is sewn into the medial side of the latissimus tendon to complete the "cuffing" of tissue over the humeral head. The deltoid is then closed as previously described and the latissimus incision is closed over drains. The shoulder is immobilized on an abduction orthosis to maintain the arm in a position of abduction and external rotation. The repair and position of immobilization are chosen so that the tendon transfer will heal under some tension and thus give a passive tenodesis effect that probably acts to keep the humeral head on the glenoid in early ranges of abduction.

Postoperative Care
Passive motion from this position of abduction is begun on the first day after surgery and continues for 6 weeks. The abduction pillow is then removed, and the patient begins active-assisted range of motion. An effort is made to retrain the latissimus to act as a humeral head depressor. To do this the therapist attempts to teach the patient to fire the latissimus at the initiation of abduction and flexion by having the patient adduct the slightly flexed arm toward the sagittal plane when initiating flexion. The latissimus will then contract as the deltoid begins to elevate the arm. Gradually the latissimus will be able to contract with the arm closer to abduction.

Recently, I found that cutaneous biofeedback training using a unit with an audible and visible signal may increase the success of this type of muscle retraining. The time course for recovery of shoulder flexion so that the patient can raise the arm above the horizontal may be up to 1 year.

Outcome of Latissimus Dorsi Transfer
Gerber's experience[26] in 16 cases with a 3-year follow-up was that forward flexion improved from a mean of 83° to 135°. Overall, 24 of the 50 patients who he treated for a massive rotator cuff tear required a latissimus transfer.

Aoki and associates[79] reported on 12 cases of irreparable rotator cuff repair treated with latissimus transfer with an average follow-up of 36 months. They had good to excellent results in eight and fair to poor results in four. The average improvement in forward flexion was from 99° to 135°. Both Gerber and Aoki and associates demonstrated by electromyographic analysis that the majority of tendon transfers are dynamic.

My (JPW) personal experience has been with 22 cases of latissimus dorsi transfer performed over a 5-year period. Results have been variable, with seven good to excellent, seven fair, and eight poor (Fig. 50). Poor results tended to occur in patients who had preexistent arthritis, deltoid deficiency from prior surgery, obesity, and poor compliance with the posteroperative therapy program.

ANTERIOR-SUPERIOR ROTATOR CUFF TEARS: SUBSCAPULARIS AND SUPRASPINATUS

EPIDEMIOLOGY/MECHANISM OF INJURY

This configuration of rotator cuff tear consists of variable lesions involving the supraspinatus, subscapularis, biceps tendon, and the coracohumeral and glenohumeral ligaments. Typically, this configuration of rotator cuff tear affects predominantly men in their fifth or sixth decade of life, and about 85% are caused by a specific trauma.[80,81] This etiology distinguishes these tears from the posterior-superior configuration of rotator cuff tear in which attritional disease of the rotator cuff is a more common etiology. The mechanism of injury is usually a sudden external rotation or hyperextension force applied to the shoulder with the arm close to the side.[80,82] If an individual older than 40 years of age reports such a mechanism of injury, or if he reports a traumatic anterior dislocation, a lesion of the subscapularis should specifically be ruled out.

There are several important points to emphasize about these kinds of rotator cuff tears. First, anterosuperior lesions of the rotator cuff have a different clinical presentation and prognosis than posterosuperior tears, and thus should be considered separately. Second, recognition both preoperatively and intraoperatively may not be straightforward, and thus there is a relative risk of missing this diagnosis. Third, treatment is difficult and the prognosis is generally less favorable than that for treatment of posterior-superior tears of the rotator cuff. Standardized treatment guidelines only recently have been presented in the literature.[81–83]

In general, acute cases of subscapularis rupture usually have tendon tissue of good quality, and surgical mobilization and repair is technically straightforward. Conversely, chronic ruptures of the subscapularis have tendon tissue of poor quality, and in this situation there is actually loss of tendon substance and scarring and retraction of the tear underneath the axillary nerve and brachial plexus. Surgical dissection and repair are difficult and fraught with risk to the neurovascular structures. As a general rule, the prognosis after surgical treatment correlates with the chronicity of the conditions.

ANATOMY OF THE ANTEROSUPERIOR ROTATOR CUFF

This region is composed of the supraspinatus and subscapularis tendons, and the components of the rotator interval that include the coracohumeral and glenohumeral ligaments and the long head of the biceps brachii. The subscapularis muscle is a large muscle that originates on the anterior scapula and makes up about 40% of the cross-sectional area of the rotator cuff. Its upper two thirds forms a relatively discrete and robust tendon, which inserts on the upper border of the lesser tuberosity, and which also conjoins with the supraspinatus tendon to form a fibrous arch over the anterior-superior region of the shoulder in the area of the rotator interval. The inferior one third of the subscapularis is mostly muscular at its insertion on the lesser tuberosity. The coracohumeral and superior glenohumeral ligaments are the main ligamentous components of the rotator interval, and together they insert into the upper lesser tuberosity and anterior portion of the greater tuberosity. These ligaments along with the subscapularis form the medial wall of the soft-tissue support for the long head of the biceps in its bicipital groove. Medial subluxation of the long head of biceps, thus, cannot occur without disruption of these structures.

CLINICAL PRESENTATION

Patients may present with several different types of complaints. About 50% of patients present with pain after a specific traumatic event. They may have good function, but have pain at night as well as pain when the shoulder is used in adduction and external rotation. There may be associated complaints referrable to the long head of the biceps tendon, because injury to this structure often accompanies subscapularis pathology. Typically, the patient may have the sensation of snapping in the front of the shoulder with external rotation as the long head of biceps subluxates intra-articularly.

Some patients may present with profound shoulder weakness with or without marked pain. These individuals have a form of pseudoparalysis with preserved passive range of motion but poor active motion. They may or may not remember a traumatic event, and they usually have near global involvement of the rotator cuff with three or more tendons disrupted.

DIAGNOSIS: IMPORTANT POINTS AND PITFALLS

Physical examination for this condition may be very sensitive and specific, and several points should be emphasized. Although active flexion and abduction may be quite good, these patients often have the appearance of anterior-superior subluxation of the humeral head. This observation can be brought out by standing behind a seated patient and having the patient attempt abduction against resistance (Fig. 52). The humeral head on the symptomatic side will be seen to move anteriorly and superiorly. Involvement of the supraspinatus can be confirmed by a positive external rotation lag sign when tested with the arm in adduction[50] and a positive supraspinatus test,[84] which is weakness and pain when the patient resists abduction of the internally rotated shoulder. Many patients will also have findings consistent with biceps injury or subluxation. These include point tenderness over the bicipital groove and positive biceps stretch or tension tests, including Speed's test (resisted flexion of the shoulder with the arm supinated and the elbow extended)[85] and Yerguson's test[86] (shoulder pain with resisted supination of the hand).

Four physical findings are pathognomonic for subscapularis tears[80,81,87] (Fig. 39). These patients have (1) painful apprehension against external rotation of the adducted shoulder; (2) a passive increase in external rotation with the arm in adduction compared to the other side (Fig. 53, *A*); (3) weakness of internal rotation strength (Fig. 53, *B*); and (4) a positive "lift-off" sign (Figs. 53, *C* and *D*). The lift-off test is performed by having the patient

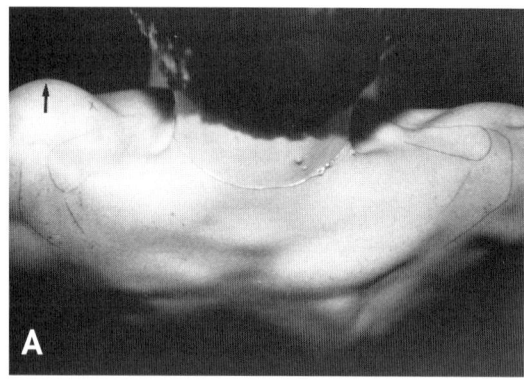 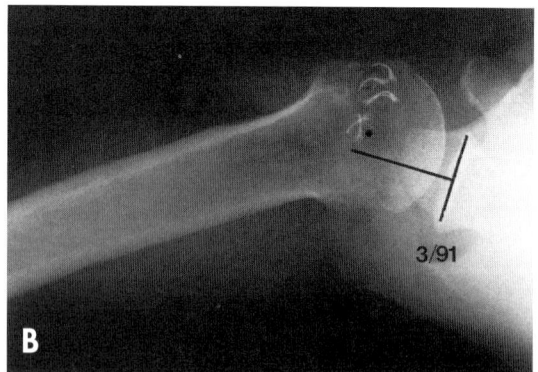

FIGURE 52

A, Patient with a anterior-superior subluxation of the humeral head in the setting of a subscapularis-supraspinatus tendon tear. (Courtesy of Christian Gerber, MD, Zurich, Switzerland.) **B,** An axillary radiograph shows static anterior subluxation in a patient with a chronic subscapularis and supraspinatus tear. (Reproduced with permission from Ticker JB, Warner JJP: Single-tendon tears of the rotator cuff: Evaluation and treatment of subscapularis tears and principles of treatment for supraspinatus tears. *Orthop Clin North Am* 1997;28:99–116.)

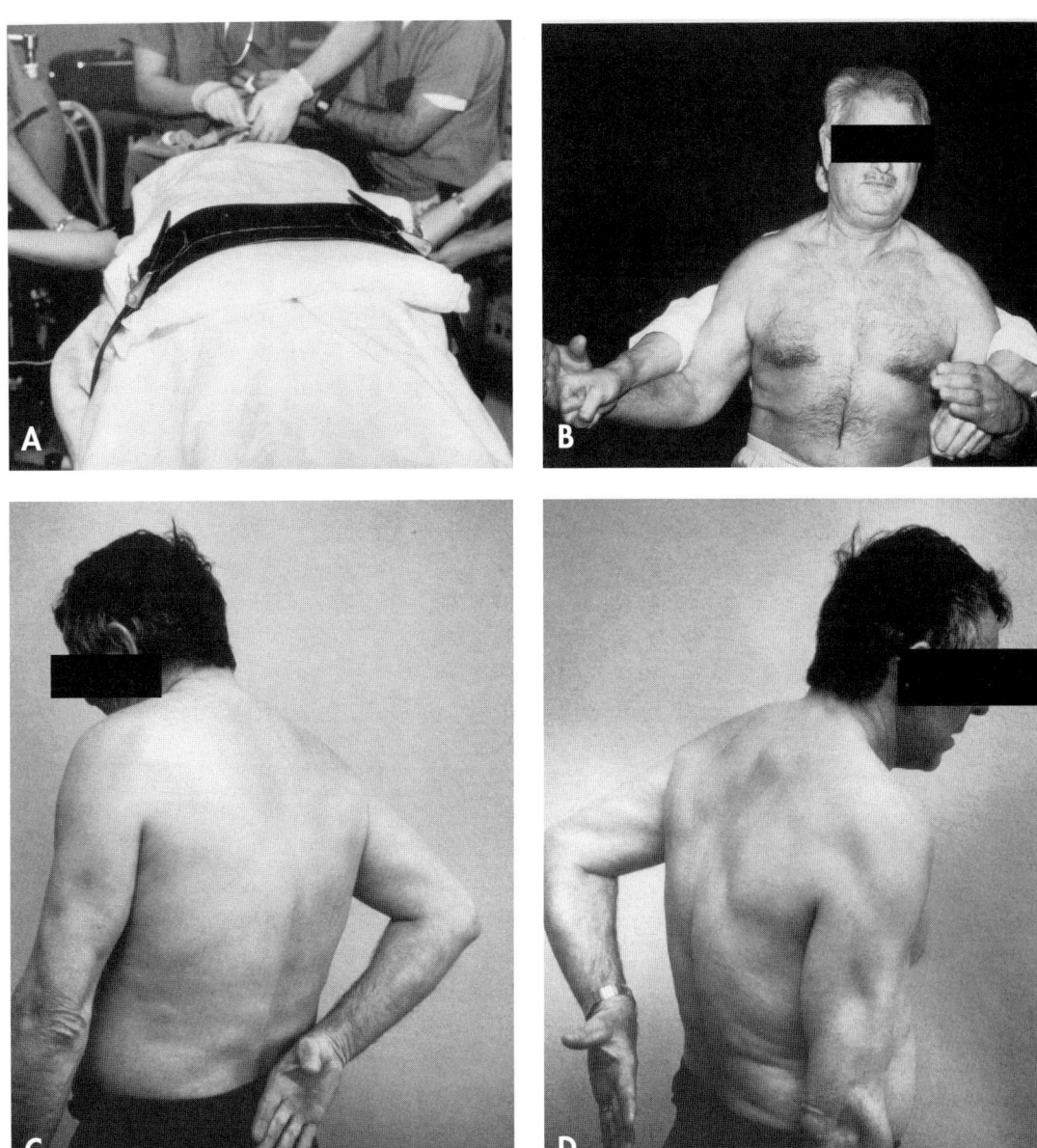

FIGURE 53

Physical findings of subscapularis tendon tear. **A,** Increased passive external rotation of the adducted shoulder. **B,** Weak internal rotation strength. **C** and **D,** Positive "lift-off" test on the right side compared with normal left side. (Reproduced with permission from Ticker JB, Warner JJP: Single-tendon tears of the rotator cuff: Evaluation and treatment of subscapularis tears and principles of treatment for supraspinatus tears. *Orthop Clin North Am* 1997;28:99–116.)

internally rotate the arm so that the hand rests on the lower back or buttock. The patient is then asked to lift the hand off the back without extending the elbow. Normal subscapularis function is required because this motion represents the end-range of internal rotation. The modified lift-off sign (Figs. 53, *E* and *F*) is a more sensitive alternative. In this test the patient's arm is internally rotated passively by the examiner into a position of maximum internal rotation, and then the patient is asked to maintain the hand in that position. A positive test will be seen as failure to maintain this arm position because the shoulder falls back into external rotation. In some patients there is limitation of internal rotation, and in these situations the lift-off sign cannot be performed. Another means of testing subscapularis function in these individuals is with the "belly-press" test.[83,87] The patient is asked to place his or her hand on his or her abdomen and, while keeping the elbow forward, to push against the abdomen. The examiner can place his or her hand between the patient's abdomen and hand in order to palpate the force of internal rotation when the patient is asked to push against his or her abdomen. A normal test will be good internal rotation strength with the patient able to keep the elbow forward. A positive test, which indicates a subscapularis tear, will be weak internal rotation with the elbow moving posteriorly when the patient tries to push his or her hand against his or her abdomen.

IMAGING STUDIES

Plain radiographs are usually helpful only in ruling out other conditions of an osseous nature, such as fractures. Occasionally several helpful findings may be identified that are specific for subscapularis disruption. These include cystic changes in the lesser tuberosity and anterior subluxation on the axillary lateral radiograph (Fig. 52, *B*).

Arthrography may be helpful in identification of an associated supraspinatus tendon tear; how-

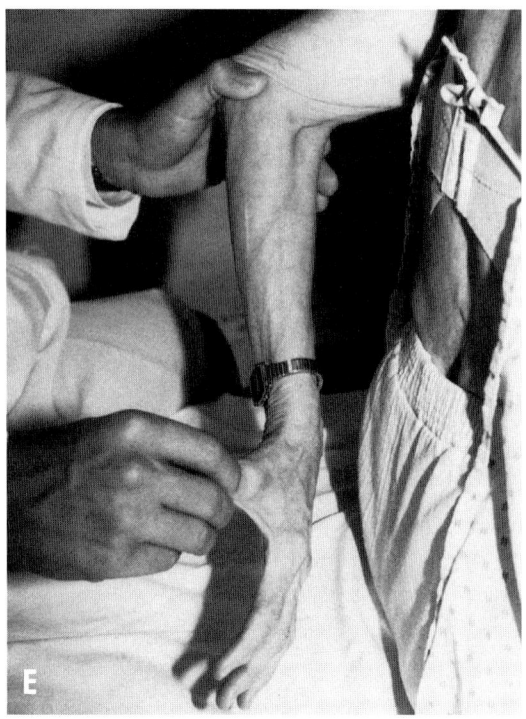 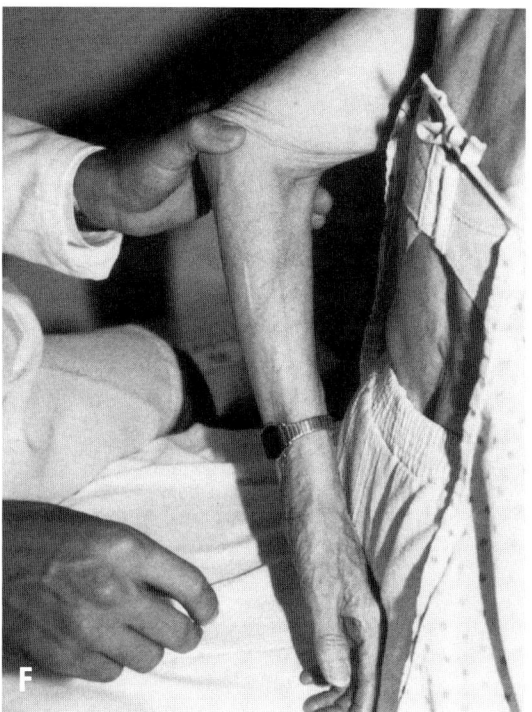

FIGURE 53 (CONTINUED)
Physical findings of subscapularis tendon tear. **E** and **F**, Positive "lift-off" sign. (Reproduced with permission from Warner JJP, Allen AA, Gerber C: Diagnosis and management of subscapularis tendon tears. *Tech Orthop* 1994;9:116–125).

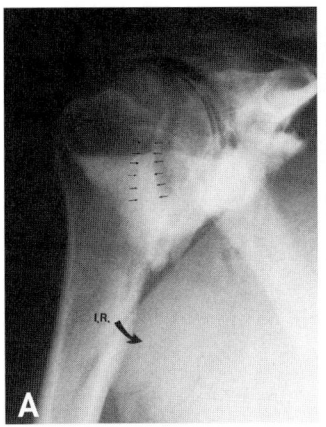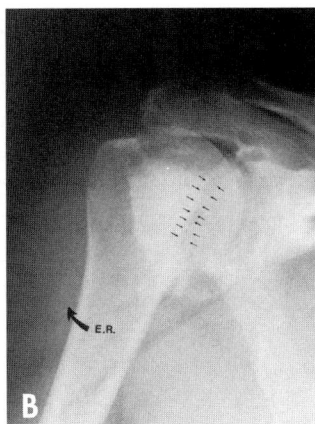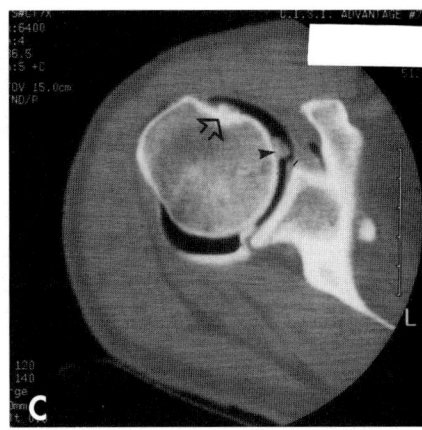

FIGURE 54
A, Biceps tendon (small arrows) outline on arthrogram with the shoulder in internal rotation (IR). **B,** With the shoulder in external rotation (ER) the biceps tendon remains medially subluxated (small arrows) as the lesser tuberosity moves laterally. **C,** CT arthrogram shows medially subluxated biceps tendon (solid arrow) with dye transmission across the lesser tuberosity (open arrow) in this patient with a subscapularis tear and medial biceps tendon subluxation. (Reproduced with permission from Ticker JB, Warner JJP: Single-tendon tears of the rotator cuff: Evaluation and treatment of subscapularis tears and principles of treatment for supraspinatus tears. *Orthop Clin North Am* 1997;28:99–116.)

ever, findings of a subscapularis tear may be subtle. If the subscapularis is torn and the long head of the biceps tendon is subluxated, the arthrogram may demonstrate that the long head of the biceps tendon remains in a medially subluxated position even when the shoulder is externally rotated (Fig. 54, *A* and *B*).

Computed tomography and MRI may both be quite sensitive and specific, especially if intra-articular dye enhancement is used.[82,83] In either test, complete subscapularis rupture will be shown by transmission of dye across the lesser tuberosity and into the bicipital groove, and a medially subluxated biceps tendon may also be demonstrated (Fig. 54, *C*). MRI may also demonstrate partial subscapularis ruptures as well. Finally, MRI is particularly helpful in providing information about the quality and quantity of subscapularis muscle (Fig. 55). This information is useful in determining the prognosis of treatment.[41]

Arthroscopy may occasionally be helpful in equivocal cases; however, careful physical examination and technically good MRI-arthrogram study will have a very high degree of sensitivity for even partial subscapularis tears.[80–83]

SURGICAL TECHNIQUE: PRIMARY CASES

Patient Positioning
The patient is positioned on a long bean bag in an upright seated position with the head of the bed at about a 45° angle. The bean bag is then contoured so that the front and back of the shoulder are free and the head is supported. I (JPW) use a special sterile articulated arm holder (McConnell Shoulder Holder; McConnell Orthopaedics, Greenville, TX) to support and position the arm.

Surgical Approach
The standard anterior-superior incision used to repair a supraspinatus-infraspinatus tendon tear may be adequate for acute tears that involve the supraspinatus and the upper half of the subscapularis; however, complete avulsion of the subscapularis is most safely and effectively treated through an anterior deltopectoral approach. This approach permits careful identification and mobilization of the axillary nerve and brachial plexus, which is a mandatory step, especially in the case of a chronic subscapularis tendon tear.

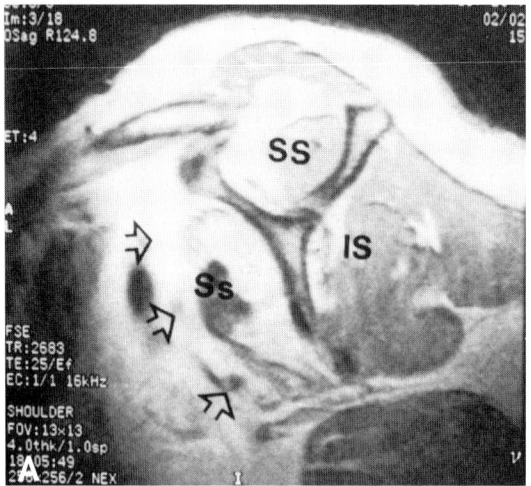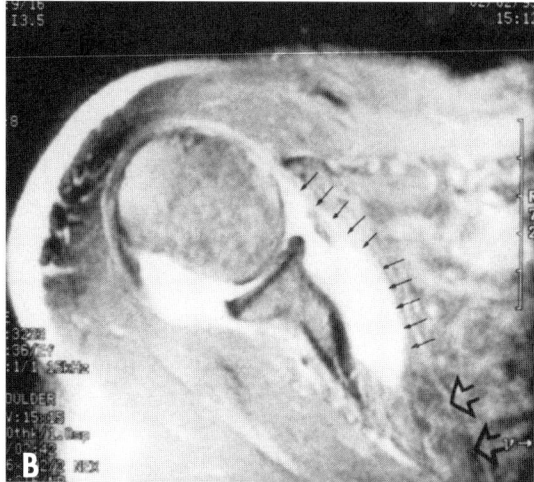

FIGURE 55

Magnetic resonance image (MRI) of a patient with a chronic subscapularis and supraspinatus tendon rupture. **A,** Oblique-saggital image demonstrates fatty replacement of the subscapularis (Ss). The supraspinatus (SS) is also mostly fat while the infraspinatus (IS) muscle has only mild fatty degeneration. **B,** MRI with gadolinium dye in a patient with a chronic subscapularis tear. There is some loss of tendon and muscle with the dye tracking into the subscapularis fossa (arrows). (Reproduced with permission from Ticker JB, Warner JJP: Single-tendon tears of the rotator cuff: Evaluation and treatment of subscapularis tears and principles of treatment for supraspinatus tears. *Orthop Clin North Am* 1997;28:99–116.)

If an individual has a combined subscapularis-supraspinatus tear pattern, an attempt is made to repair both through a deltopectoral incision, although tears that extend superiorly and posteriorly may require extension of the incision superiorly with formal deltoid detachment and splitting (Fig. 56).

The subscapularis tendon often remains in continuity with the lesser tuberosity through a thin, tapered extension of scar or bursa, and the biceps tendon can sometimes be seen to be subluxated underneath this tissue when the shoulder is externally rotated (Fig. 57). This injury is really a disinsertion with scar in continuity rather than an avulsion. When this thin scar is detached from the lesser tuberosity, it can be traced medially to the retracted bulk of the subscapularis tendon. In most cases the superior two thirds of the tendon is torn, and the muscular component of the inferior tendon remains attached to the lesser tuberosity.

The degree of mobilization and dissection is dictated by the amount of retraction of the tendon and the chronicity of the tear (Fig. 58, *A* and *B*). In acute tendon tears, the edge of the tendon can be identified and reinserted into the lesser tuberosity without need for extensive releases. However, in chronic tendon tears, extensive dissection and release may be necessary before repair of the subscapularis is possible.

In these cases, once the residual soft tissue is detached from the lesser tuberosity, a humeral head retractor is inserted into the joint in order to push the humeral head posteriorly. This will greatly improve the ease of dissection anteriorly. Sutures are then placed in the edge of the tendon tear and tension is applied through these sutures as the tendon is mobilized and released. A long, thin retractor is then inserted underneath the conjoined tendon and the brachial plexus and axillary nerve are identified (Fig. 58, *C* and *D*). The axillary nerve is mobilized, and a vessel loupe is placed around it so that it can be protected during the remainder of the dissection. The subscapularis tendon is usually retracted medially and inferiorly, so adhesions must be released in this plane. Scissors are used to divide along the inferior border of the subscapularis tendon, releasing it from the underlying capsule. This division is carried medially underneath the axillary nerve which is protected with an elevator or

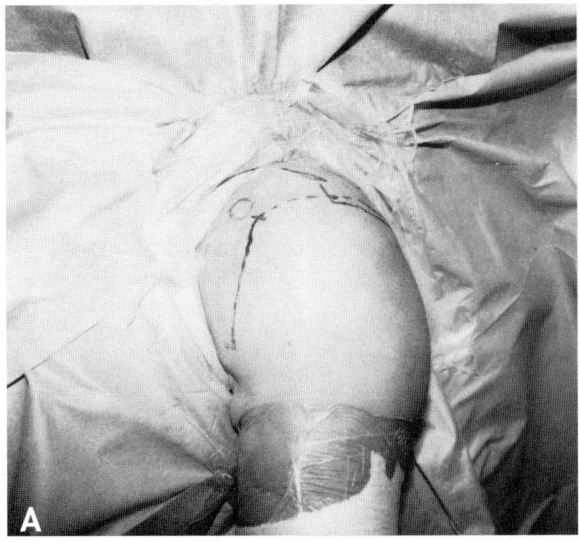
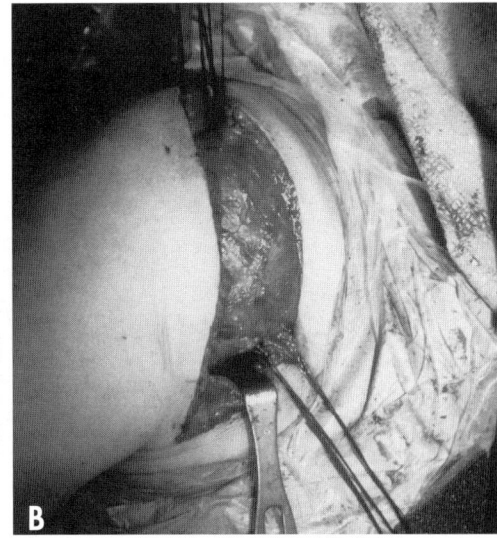

FIGURE 56

Authors' prefered surgical approach for patients with massive anterior-superior rotator cuff tears. **A,** The incision is in the anterior axillary line, as for a deltopectoral exposure, and continues over the top of the acromion. **B,** The deltoid is only partially detached from the acromion so surgery is performed through a deltopectoral approach (for subscapularis repair) and lateral deltoid split approach (for supraspinatus).

retractor. The subscapularis is then isolated from the capsule by incising the capsule just over the anterior labrum. An elevator is then inserted into the subscapularis fossa to free up the muscle. Any scar tissue connecting the subscapularis to the base of the coracoid process is released as well. At completion of these steps, the subscapularis has been globally mobilized (Fig. 58, *C* and *D*). In most cases, this surgical dissection will give sufficient tissue so that the tendon can be reinserted into the lesser tuberosity when the arm is in neutral rotation or some degree of external rotation.

Although suture anchors can be used to repair the tendon, I (JPW) prefer instead to fashion a shallow bony trough slightly medial to the lesser tuberosity and then perform a soft tissue to bone repair with a transosseous technique as described in the preceding text (Fig. 58, *E*). If the biceps tendon is subluxated it is also usually markedly frayed. In these cases it is not recentered and repaired into the biciptial groove, but instead it is tenodesed to the humerus inferior and medial to the bicipital groove.

If the patient has extension of the tear into the supraspinatus and infraspinatus that cannot be adequately mobilized by this deltopectoral approach, the incision is extended proximally over the top of the acromion and an anterior-superior

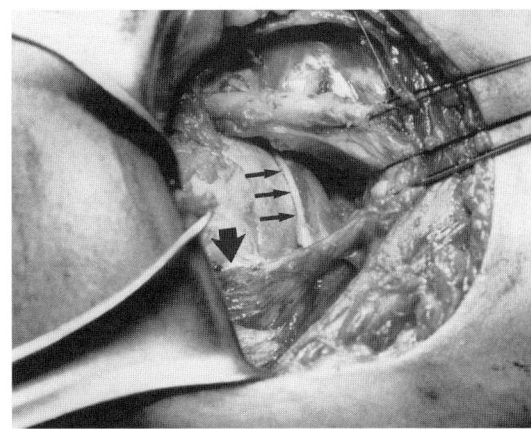

FIGURE 57

Subscapularis tendon tear with residual subluxation of the biceps tendon. Sutures have been placed through the upper two thirds of the tendon. The lower one third of the subscapularis remains attached to the lesser tuberosity (large arrow). The biceps tendon is subluxated medially (small arrows). (Reproduced with permission from Warner JJP, Allen AA, Gerber C: Diagnosis and management of subscapularis tendon tears. *Tech Orthop* 1994;9:116–125.)

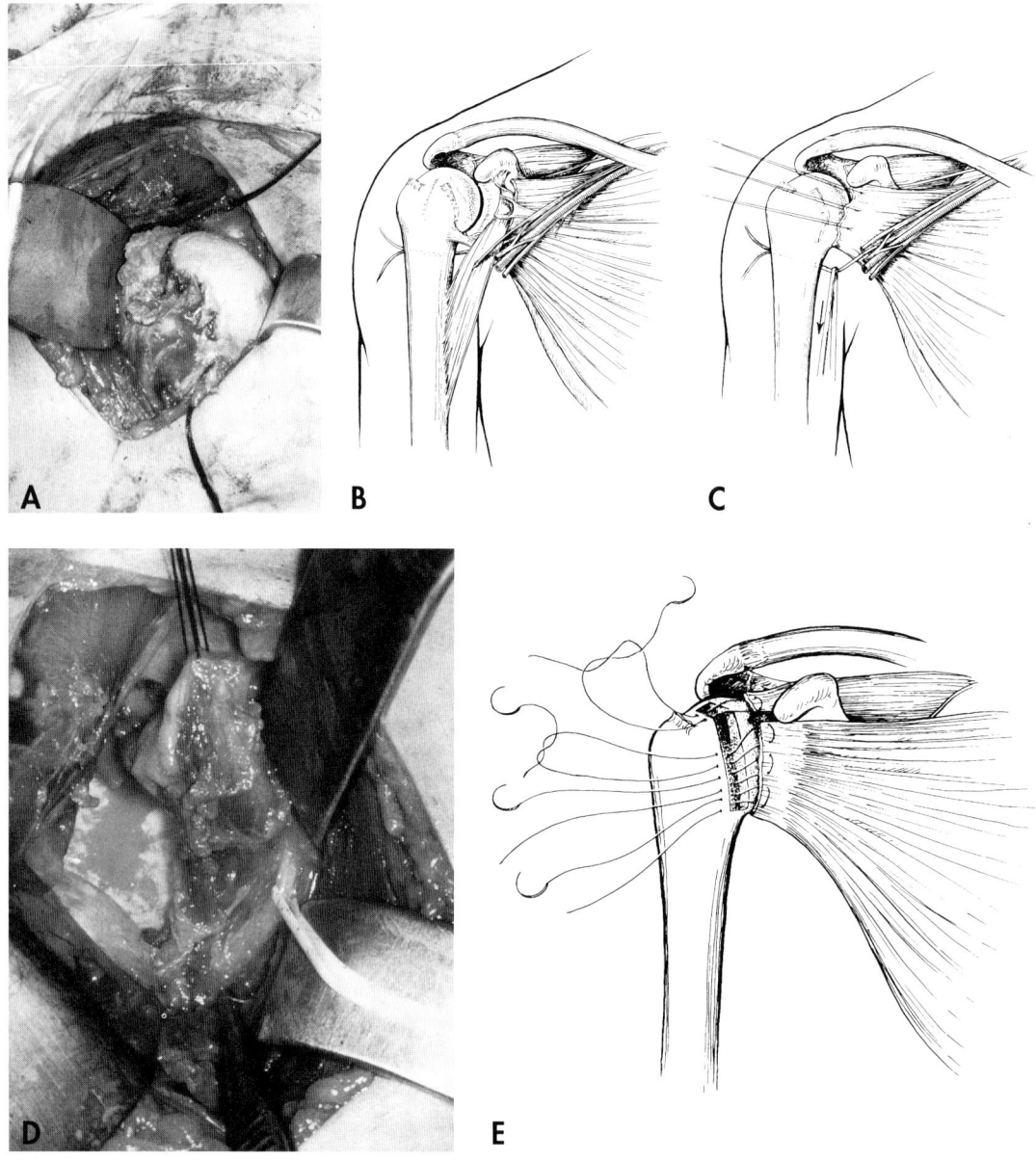

FIGURE 58

Technique of subscapularis and supraspinatus tendon repair. **A** and **B,** Retracted tear of the upper three-fourths of the subscapularis tendon. Note the proximity of the neurovascular structures. **C** and **D,** Axillary nerve dissection and mobilization of the subscapularis tendon. **E,** Transosseous repair of the subscapularis and supraspinatus. (Reproduced with permission from Warner JJP, Allen AA, Gerber C: Diagnosis and management of subscapularis tendon tears. *Tech Orthop* 1994;9:116–125.)

approach with detachment of a portion of the deltoid is performed (Figs. 56 and 58, *C*). The infraspinatus and supraspinatus tendons are then mobilized and repaired as described previously.

POSTOPERATIVE TREATMENT

The ranges for passive motion are determined based on the intraoperative observation of the tension on the repair site. Aggressive external rotation is not permitted for the first 6 weeks. Patients are also instructed to avoid any forceful use of the arm or heavy lifting until 6 to 8 months after surgery.

CLINICAL RESULTS

Recent summary of a European experience with these conditions was given by Gerber and Rippensten (unpublished data, 1992) at the International Conference of Surgery of the Shoulder. Eighty-eight cases of combined supraspinatus-subscapularis tears were identified from seven centers in Europe, and it was concluded that the prevalence of this lesion and results of surgical treatment varied. Overall, the prognosis was worse than in cases of posterior-superior tendon tears treated surgically. All cases had concomitant biceps tendon pathology, and only 25% were able to achieve forward flexion greater than 150° after surgical treatment.

Frankle and Cofield (unpublished data, 1992) identified 24 subscapularis-supraspinatus tendon tears out of 301 rotator cuff surgeries performed over a period of 5 years, and all of these also had biceps tendon pathology. The average forward flexion achieved after surgery was 134°, and 25% of these patients had significant weakness and pain.

Recently, Gerber and associates[87] presented their results for surgical treatment of 16 subscapularis ruptures. With an average follow-up of 43 months, they found that active forward flexion was normal or near normal in 15 of 16 cases, and that most patients recovered the capacity to participate in their preinjury level of employment. The single most important factor in determination of outcome was the length of delay from time of injury to time of surgical repair.

SURGICAL TECHNIQUE: REVISIONS CASES

Definition of "Irreparable"

There is little available information on the inci-dence of irreparable anterior-superior tendon tears and the option for management of this difficult problem. The problematic component of the tear is usually the subscapularis rupture. The authors have a combined experience of over 100 subscapularis tendon ruptures treated surgically, and only five were described as irreparable. Wirth and associates[88] described 12 patients with irreparable subscapularis tendon tears out of 182 shoulders undergoing surgery for recurrent anterior shoulder instability. However, the criteria for determination that the tendon tear was irreparable were not well-defined. My (JPW) own definition would be that extensive tendon mobilization by the previously described techniques does not yield tendon tissue that can be repaired to the lesser tuberosity with the arm in neutral rotation. These kinds of problems usually occur in patients with long-standing subscapularis tendon tears, with severe fatty replacement of the muscle on MRI, or with prior failed attempts at repair of the subscapularis.

Surgical Treatment Options

Contrary to posterior-superior tendon tears, there are few options for tendon transfer to substitute for loss of subscapularis function. Pectoralis major or minor tendon transfer has been suggested as an alternative method of treatment; however, it is difficult to understand how this transfer can substitute for the function of the subscapularis, because the vector of the pectoralis major is anterior relative to the center of rotation of the humeral head, whereas the subscapularis vector is posteriorly directed (Fig. 59). Nevertheless, Wirth and associates[88] described transfer of these tendons in their 12 patients and nine (82%) had a satisfactory result while two (18%) had an unsatisfactory result. The experience of shoulder surgeons in Europe has been less favorable. My (JPW) experience with two cases using a modified pectoralis major transfer has been satisfactory. The technique transfers the sternal head of the pectoralis major underneath its clavicular head so that it is inserted into the lesser tuberosity (Fig. 59). Both patients have had decrease in their pain and elimination of instability with a short-term follow-up.

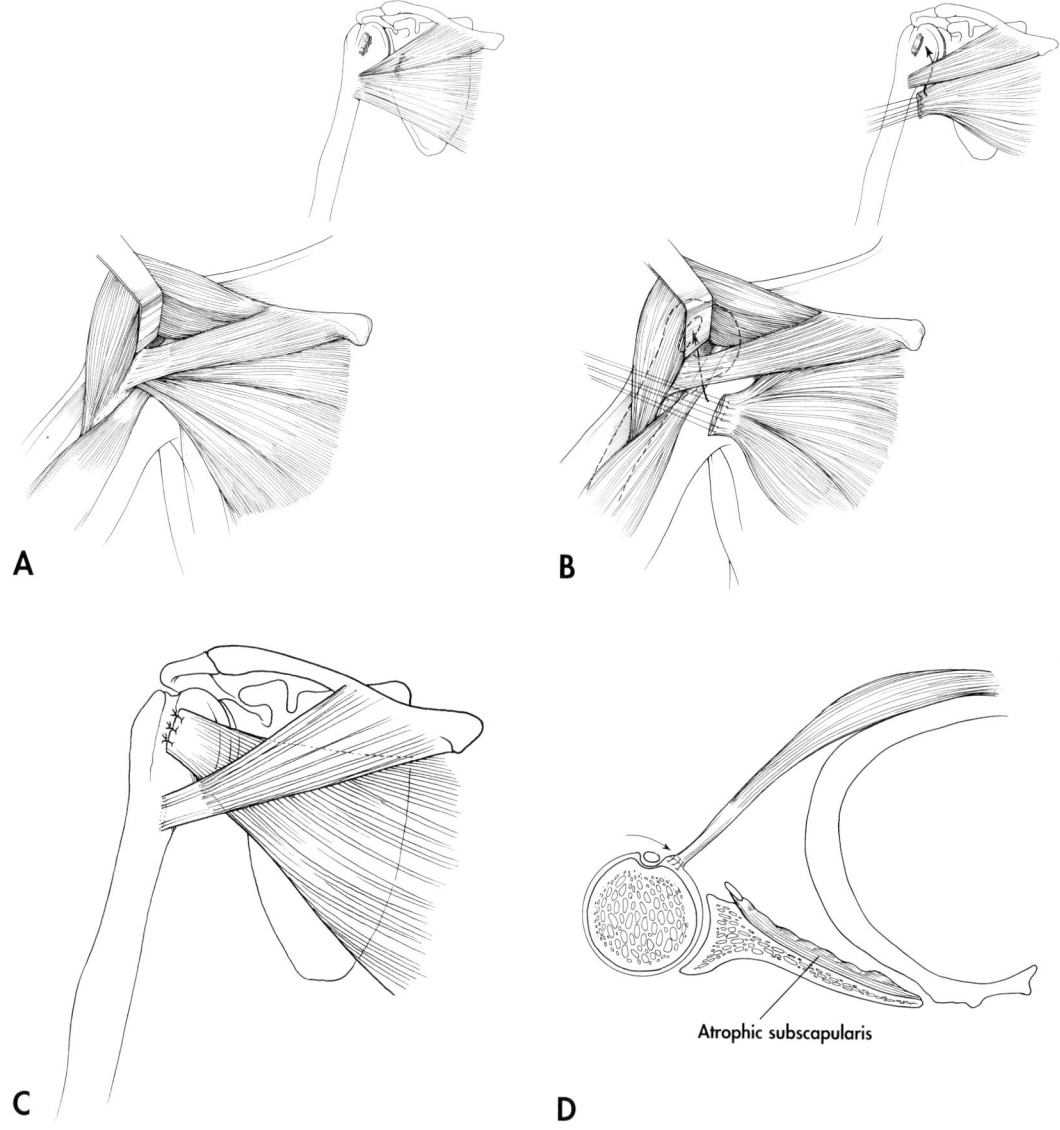

A

B

C

D

Atrophic subscapularis

FIGURE 59
Technique of pectoralis major reconstruction of subscapularis tendon.

SUMMARY

Although massive rotator cuff tears are uncommon, their treatment remains a difficult challenge. Recognition of the difference between posterior-superior and anterior-superior tear configurations is important because treatment approaches and prognosis differ between these two entities. Careful preoperative evaluation based on physical examination and adjuvant imaging studies will allow the physician to identify those patients who have good tendon quality and an overall good prognosis, as well as those who have poor tendon quality and a poor prognosis. The MRI appearance of the rotator cuff musculature is a particularly helpful observation because tendon quality and recovery of overall function may be correlated with the degree of atrophy and fatty replacement by the muscle. In general, patients with acute tendon tears and minimal fatty replacement and muscle atrophy have a good prognosis. Conversely, patients with chronic loss of function and an MRI that demonstrates fatty replacement and muscle atrophy have a poor prognosis. Revision techniques such as latissimus dorsi tendon transfer may be very useful in select patients with irreparable rotator cuff tears.

REFERENCES

1. Neer CS II (ed): Cuff tears, biceps lesions, and impingement, in *Shoulder Reconstruction.* Philadelphia, PA, WB Saunders, 1990, pp 41–142.

2. Bigliani LU, Cordasco FA, McIlveen SJ, Musso ES: Operative repair of massive rotator cuff tears: Long-term results. *J Shoulder Elbow Surg* 1992;1:120–130.

3. Ellman H, Hanker G, Bayer M: Repair of the rotator cuff: End result study of factors influencing reconstruction. *J Bone Joint Surg* 1986;68A: 1135–1144.

4. Harryman DR II, Mack LA, Wang KY, Jackins SE, Richardson ML, Matsen FA III: Repairs of the rotator cuff: Correlation of functional results with integrity of the cuff. *J Bone Joint Surg* 1991;73A:982–989.

5. Hawkins RJ, Misamore GW, Hobeika PE: Surgery for full-thickness rotator cuff tears. *J Bone Joint Surg* 1985;67A:1345–1355.

6. Cofield RH: Rotator cuff disease of the shoulder. *J Bone Joint Surg* 1985;67A:974–979.

7. Gerber C, Vinh TS, Hertel R, Hess CW: Latissimus dorsi transfer for the treatment of massive tears of the rotator cuff: A preliminary report. *Clin Orthop* 1988;232:51–61.

8. Gschwend N, Ivosevic-Radovanovic D, Patte D: Rotator cuff tear: Relationship between clinical and anatomopathological findings. *Arch Orthop Trauma* Surg 1988;107:7–15.

9. Cofield RH: Tears of rotator cuff, in Murray DG (ed): American Academy of Orthopaedic Surgeons *Instructional Course Lectures Volume XXX.* St. Louis, MO, CV Mosby, 1981, pp 258–273.

10. Keating JF, Waterworth P, Shaw-Dunn J, Crossan J: The relative strengths of the rotator cuff muscles: A cadaver study. *J Bone Joint Surg* 1993;75B:137–140.

11. Bassett RWW, Browne AO, Morrey BF, An KN: Glenohumeral muscle force and moment mechanics in a position of shoulder instability. *J Biomech* 1990;23:405–415.

12. McMahon PJ, Debski RE, Thompson WO, Warner JJ, Fu FH, Woo SL: Shoulder muscle forces and tendon excursions during glenohumeral abduction in the scapular plane. *J Shoulder Elbow Surg* 1995;4:199–208.

13. Inman VT, Saunders JB, Abbott LC: Observations on the function of the shoulder joint. *J Bone Joint Surg* 1944;26:1–30.

14. Poppen NK, Walker PS: Forces at the glenohumeral joint in abduction. *Clin Orthop* 1978;135:165–170.

15. Bernageau J: Roentgenographic assessment of the rotator cuff. *Clin Orthop* 1990;254:87–91.

16. LeClerq R: Diagnostique de la rupture du sousepineoux. *Rev Rheum* 1950;10:510–515.

17. Watson M: Major ruptures of the rotator cuff: The results of surgical repair in 89 patients. *J Bone Joint Surg* 1985;67B:618–624.

18. Weiner DS, Macnab I: Superior migration of the humeral head: A radiological aid in the diagnosis of tears of the rotator cuff. *J Bone Joint Surg* 1970;52B:524–527.

19. Itoi E, Kuechle DK, Newman SR, Morrey BF, An KN: Stabilising function of the biceps in stable and unstable shoulders. *J Bone Joint Surg* 1993;75B:546–550.

20. Kumar VP, Satku K, Balasubramaniam P: The role of the long head of biceps brachii in the stabilization of the head of the humerus. *Clin Orthop* 1989;244:172–175.

21. Warner JJ, McMahon PJ: The role of the long head of the biceps brachii in superior stability of the glenohumeral joint. *J Bone Joint Surg* 1995;77A:355–372.

22. Burkhart SS: Reconciling the paradox of rotator cuff repair versus debridement: A unified biomechanical rationale for the treatment of rotator cuff tears. *Arthroscopy* 1994;10:4–19.

23. Burkhart SS: Arthroscopic debridement and decompression for selected rotator cuff tears: Clinical results, pathomechanics, and patient selection based on biomechanical parameters. *Orthop Clin North Am* 1993;24:111–123.

24. Rockwood CA Jr, Burkhead WZ: Management of patients with massive rotator cuff defects by acromioplasty and rotator cuff debridement. *Orthop Trans* 1988;12:190–191.

25. Thompson WO, Debski RE, Boardman ND III, et al: A biomechanical analysis of rotator cuff deficiency in a cadaveric model. *Am J Sports Med* 1996;24:286–292.

26. Gerber C: Latissimus dorsi transfer for the treatment of irreparable tears of the rotator cuff. *Clin Orthop* 1992;275:152–160.

27. Arntz CT, Matsen FA III, Jackins S: Surgical management of complex irreparable rotator cuff deficiency. *J Arthroplasty* 1991;6:353–370.

28. Bassett RW, Cofield RH: Acute tears of the rotator cuff: The timing of surgical repair. *Clin Orthop* 1983;175:18–24.

29. Bjorkenheim JM, Paavolainen P, Ahovuo J, Slatis P: Surgical repair of the rotator cuff and surrounding tissues: Factors influencing the results. *Clin Orthop* 1988;236:148–153.

30. Cofield RH: Subscapular muscle transposition for repair of chronic rotator cuff tears. *Surg Gynecol Obstet* 1982;154:667–672.

31. Debeyre J, Patte D, Elmelik E: Repair of ruptures of the rotator cuff of the shoulder: With a note on advancement of the supraspinatus muscle. *J Bone Joint Surg* 1965;47B:36–42.

32. DeOrio JK, Cofield RH: Results of a second attempt at surgical repair of a failed initial rotator cuff repair. *J Bone Joint Surg* 1984;66A:563–567.

33. Ha'eri GB, Wiley AM: Advancement of the supraspinatus muscle in the repair of ruptures of the rotator cuff. *J Bone Joint Surg* 1981;63A:232–238.

34. McLaughlin HL: Lesions of the musculotendinous cuff of the shoulder: I. The exposure and treatment of tears with retraction. *J Bone Joint Surg* 1944;26B:31–51.

35. Neviaser JS, Neviaser RJ, Neviaser TJ: The repair of chronic massive ruptures of the rotator cuff of the shoulder by use of a freeze-dried rotator cuff. *J Bone Joint Surg* 1978;60A:681–685.

36. Neviaser RJ, Neviaser TJ: Transfer of subscapularis and teres minor for massive defects of the rotator cuff, in Bayley I, Kessel L (eds): *Shoulder Surgery*. Berlin, Germany, Springer-Verlag, 1982, pp 60–63.

37. Neviaser RJ, Neviaser TJ, Neviaser JS: Concurrent rupture of the rotator cuff and anterior dislocation of the shoulder in the older patient. *J Bone Joint Surg* 1988;70A:1308–1311.

38. Petersson C: Long-term results of rotator cuff repair, in Bayley I, Kessel L (eds): *Shoulder Surgery*. Berlin, Germany, Springer-Verlag, 1982, pp 64–69.

39. Rodosky MW, Warner JJP, Waskowitz R: Abduction biomechanics in patients with massive rotator cuff tears: A roentgenographic study. Proceedings of the 60th Annual Meeting of the American Academy of Orthopaedic Surgeons, San Francisco, CA. Rosemont, IL, American Academy of Orthopaedic Surgeons, 1993, p 457.

40. Wolfgang GL: Surgical repair of tears of the rotator cuff of the shoulder: Factors influencing the result. *J Bone Joint Surg* 1974;56A:14–26.

41. Goutallier D, Postel JM, Bernageau J, Lavau L, Voisin M-C: Fatty muscle degeneration in cuff ruptures: Pre- and postoperative evaluation by CT scan. *Clin Orthop* 1994;304:78–83.

42. Flatow EL, Soslowsky LJ, Ticker JB, Pawluk RJ, Mow VC, Bigliani LU: Excursion of the rotator cuff under the acromion: Patterns of subacromial contact. *J Shoulder Elbow Surg* 1993;2:S22.

43. Ticker JB, Bigliani LU: The coracoacromial arch and rotator cuff tendinopathy. *Sports Med Arthroscopy Rev* 1995;3:8–15.

44. Lundberg BJ: The correlation of clinical evaluation with operative findings and prognosis in rotator cuff rupture, in Bayley I, Kessel L (eds): *Shoulder Surgery*. Berlin, Germany, Springer-Verlag, 1982, pp 35–38.

45. Neer CS II: Anterior acromioplasty for the chronic impingement syndrome in the shoulder: A preliminary report. *J Bone Joint Surg* 1972;54A:41–50.

46. Rathbun JB, Macnab I: The microvascular pattern of the rotator cuff. *J Bone Joint Surg* 1970;52B:540–553.

47. Matsen FA III, Arntz CT: Rotator cuff tendon failure, in Rockwood CA Jr, Matson FA III (eds): *The Shoulder*. Philadelphia, PA, WB Saunders, 1990, pp 647–677.

48. Reeves B: Experiments on the tensile strength of the anterior capsular structures of the shoulder in man. *J Bone Joint Surg* 1968;50B:858–865.

49. Ben-Yishay A, Zuckerman JD, Gallagher M, Cuomo F: Pain inhibition of shoulder strength in patients with impingement syndrome. *Orthopedics* 1994;17:685–688.

50. Hertel R, Ballmer FT, Lambert SM, Gerber C: Lag signs in the diagnosis of rotator cuff rupture. *J Shoulder Elbow Surg* 1996;5:307–313.

51. Aoki M, Ishii S, Usui M: Clinical application for measuring the slope of the acromion, in Post M, Morrey BF, Hawkins RJ (eds): *Surgery of the Shoulder*. St. Louis, MO, Mosby-Year Book, 1990, pp 200–203.

52. Bigliani LU, Morrison DS, April EW: The morphology of the acromion and its relationship to rotator cuff tears. *Orthop Trans* 1986;10:228.

53. Bigliani LU, Ticker JB, Flatow EL, Soslowsky LJ, Mow VC: The relationship of acromial architecture to rotator cuff disease. *Clin Sports Med* 1991;10:823–838.

54. Morrison DS, Bigliani LU: The clinical significance of variations in acromial morphology. *Orthop Trans* 1987;11:234.

55. Ono K, Yamamuro T, Rockwood CA Jr: Use of a thirty-degree caudal tilt radiograph in the shoulder impingement syndrome. *J Shoulder Elbow Surg* 1992;1:246–252.

56. Bigliani LU, Norris TR, Fischer J, Neer CS: The relationship between the unfused acromial epiphysis and subacromial impingement lesions. *Orthop Trans* 1983;7:138.

57. Edelson JG, Zuckerman J, Hershkovitz I: Os acromiale: Anatomy and surgical implications. *J Bone Joint Surg* 1993;75B:551–555.

58. Mudge MK, Wood VE, Frykman GK: Rotator cuff tears associated with os acromiale. *J Bone Joint Surg* 1984;66A:427–429.

59. Iannotti JP, Zlatkin MB, Esterhai JL, Kressel HY, Dalinka MK, Sprindler KP: Magnetic resonance imaging of the shoulder: Sensitivity, specificity, and predictive value. *J Bone Joint Surg* 1991;73A:17–29.

60. Nakagaki K, Ozaki J, Tomita Y, Tamai S: Alterations in the supraspinatus muscle belly with rotator cuff tearing: Evaluation with magnetic resonance imaging. *J Shoulder Elbow Surg* 1994;3:88–93.

61. Borges AF: Relaxed skin tension lines (RSTL) versus other skin lines. *Plast Rconstr Surg* 1984;73:144–150.

62. Kraissl CJ: The selection of appropriate lines for elective surgical incisions. *Plast Reconstr Surg* 1951;8:1–28.

63. Neer CS II, Satterlee CC, Dalsey RM, Flatow EL: On the value of the coracohumeral ligament release. *Orthop Trans* 1989;13:234–236.

64. Warner JJP, Krushell RJ, Masquelet A, Gerber C: Anatomy and relationships of the suprascapular nerve: Anatomical constraints to mobilization of the supraspinatus and infraspinatus muscles in the management of massive rotator-cuff tears. *J Bone Joint Surg* 1992;74A:36–45.

65. Gerber C, Schneeberger AG, Beck M, Schlegel U: Mechanical strength of repairs of the rotator cuff. *J Bone Joint Surg* 1994;76B:371–380.

66. Calvert PT, Packer NP, Stoker DJ, Bayley JI, Kessel L: Arthrography of the shoulder after operative repair of the torn rotator cuff. *J Bone Joint Surg* 1986;68B:147–150.

67. Caldwell GL Jr, Warner JJP, Miller MD, Towers J, Debski RE: Transosseous rotator cuff fixation: The weak link? A biomechanical evaluation. Proceedings of the 62nd Annual Meeting of the American Academy of Orthopaedic Surgeons, Orlando, FL, 1995. Rosemont, IL, American Academy of Orthopaedic Surgeons, p 195.

68. France EP, Paulos LE, Harner CD, Straight CB: Biomechanical evaluation of rotator cuff fixation methods. *Am J Sports Med* 1989;17:176–181.

69. Sward L, Hughes JS, Amis A, Wallace WA: The strength of surgical repairs of the rotator cuff: A biomechanical study of cadavers. *J Bone Joint Surg* 1992;74B:585–588.

70. Stone JK, von Faunhofer JA, Massterson BJ: Mechanical properties of coated absorbable multifilament suture materials. *Obstet Gynecol* 1986;67:737–740.

71. Bourne RB, Bitar H, Andreae PR, Martin LM, Finlay JB, Marquis F: In-vivo comparison of four absorbable sutures: Vicryl, Dexon Plus, Maxon, and PDS. *Can J Surg* 1988;31:43–45.

72. Krackow KA, Thomas SC, Jones LC: A new stitch for ligament-tendon fixation: Brief note. *J Bone Joint Surg* 1986;68A:764–766.

73. Groh GI, Simoni M, Rolla P, Rockwood CA: Loss of the deltoid after shoulder operations: An operative disaster. *J Shoulder Elbow Surg* 1994;3:243–253.

74. Karas SE, Giachello TL: Subscapularis transfer for reconstruction of massive tears of the rotator cuff. *J Bone Joint Surg* 1996;78A:239–245.

75. Ellman H, Kay SP, Wirth M: Arthroscopic treatment of full-thickness rotator cuff tears: 2- to 7-year follow-up study. *Arthroscopy* 1993;9:195–200.

76. Heikel HV: Rupture of the rotator cuff of the shoulder: Experiences of surgical treatment. *Acta Orthop Scand* 1968;39:477–492.

77. Ozaki J, Fujimoto S, Masuhara K, Tamai S, Yoshimoto S: Reconstruction of chronic massive rotator cuff tears with synthetic materials. *Clin Orthop* 1986;202:173–183.

78. Post M: Rotator cuff repair with carbon filament: A preliminary report of five cases. *Clin Orthop* 19856;196:154–158.

79. Aoki M, Okamura K, Fukushima S, Takahashi T, Ogino T: Transfer of latissimus dorsi for irreparable rotator-cuff tears. *J Bone Joint Surg* 1996;78B:761–766.

80. Gerber C, Krushell RJ: Isolated rupture of the tendon of the subscapularis muscle: Clinical features in 16 cases. *J Bone Joint Surg* 1991; 73B:389–394.

81. Warner JJP, Allen AA, Gerber C: Diagnosis and management of subscapularis tendon tears. *Tech Orthop* 1994;9:1161–125.

82. Deutsch A, Altchek DW, Veltri DM, Potter HG, Warren RF: Traumatic tears of the subscapularis tendon: Clinical diagnosis, magnetic resonance imaging findings, and operative treatment. *Am J Sports Med* 1997;25:13–22.

83. Nové-Josserand L, Gerber C, Walch G: Lesions of the antero-superior rotator cuff, in Warner JJP, Iannotti JP, Gerber C (eds): *Complex and Revision Problems in Shoulder Surgery.* Philadelphia, PA, Lippincott-Raven, 1997, pp 165–176.

84. Borges AF: Relaxed skin tension lines (RSTL) versus other skin lines. *Plast Reconstr Surg* 1984;73:144–150.

85. Gilcreest EL: The common syndrome of rupture, dislocation, and elongation of the long head of the biceps brachii: An analysis of one hundred cases. *Surg Gynecol Obstet* 1934;58:322–340.

86. Yergason RM: Supination sign. *J Bone Joint Surg* 1931;13B:160.

87. Gerber C, Hersche O, Farron A: Isolated rupture of the subscapularis tendon. *J Bone Joint Surg* 1996;78A:1015–1023.

88. Wirth MA, Seltzer DG, Rockwood CA Jr: Replacement of the subscapularis with the pectoralis muscles in anterior shoulder instability. Proceedings of the 62nd Annual Meeting of the American Academy of Orthopaedic Surgeons, Orlando FL. Rosemont, IL, American Academy of Orthopaedic Surgeons, 1995, p 342.

COMPLICATIONS RELATED TO ROTATOR CUFF SURGERY

R. JOHN NARANJA, JR, MD

JOSEPH P. IANNOTTI, MD, PHD

INTRODUCTION

The management of rotator cuff tears and symptoms related to rotator cuff disease has undergone a progressive evolution since the first reported rotator cuff repair in 1911.[1] The understanding of cuff pathology has been fostered by identification of the intrinsic vulnerability of the cuff to degenerative injury secondary to its blood supply,[2] as well as the extrinsic anatomic considerations that have been shown to impinge on the cuff.[3,4] A spectrum of clinical manifestations ranging from an asymptomatic cuff tear[5] to the advancing stages of impingement—stage I, hemorrhage and edema; stage II, tendonitis and fibrosis; and stage III, full thickness tear—has been recognized.[4]

The literature has consistently indicated the ability to obtain good results from surgical treatment when conservative measures fail. A careful analysis demonstrates the pitfalls of poor patient selection, errors in technique, and complications unforeseeable by any measure of preoperative planning. Complications may be divided into those secondary to incorrect or incomplete diagnosis, those related to decompression, those related to repair, and those related to postoperative rehabilitation or wound healing difficulties.

COMPLICATIONS RELATED TO INCORRECT OR INCOMPLETE DIAGNOSIS

The diagnosis of impingement and/or symptomatic rotator cuff tear requires a complete history and physical examination and may include appropriate confirmatory tests, such as imaging, electromyographic, and laboratory studies. Impingement classically is diagnosed by pain at the anterior aspect of the shoulder, which is aggravated by forced forward elevation of the humerus against the acromion (positive impingement sign), and relief of pain after injection of 10 cc of 1% lidocaine in the subacromial space (positive impingement test). Other diagnoses that must be excluded may be classified[6] as those related to referred pain (cervical radiculitis, thoracic outlet syndrome, suprascapular nerve entrapment), intra-articular pathology (glenohumeral instability, labral tears, glenohumeral osteoarthritis), extra-articular pathology (acromioclavicular joint arthritis, adhesive capsulitis, unrecognized or untreated rotator cuff tear), and secondary gain issues (worker's compensation).

Referred pain related to cervical disk disease is a common source of misdiagnosis.[3,6–9] Cervical pathology may occur concomitantly with impingement or present alone as a cause of chronic shoulder pain. Patients' response to treatment will depend on the proportion of findings related to cervical pathology versus that attributed to impingement at the coracoacromial arch. Prognosis is more difficult to interpret for those who undergo surgery for impingement in the context of coexisting cervical disk disease.

The path of the suprascapular nerve through the confining anatomy of the suprascapular notch makes it susceptible to compression and resulting symptoms that may mimic the findings associated with a rotator cuff tear. The diagnosis must be entertained in the young patient with no history of trauma and loss of power associated with vague pain at the posterior aspect of the shoulder. Confirmation with electromyographic examination is useful. Treatment is directed at the etiology of the nerve compression.

Thoracic outlet syndrome as a cause of referred pain to the shoulder[6–8] is related to compression of the nerves and vessels to the upper limb as they exit the interval between the scalene muscles, travel over the first rib, and course down into the axilla. The history typically includes pain and paresthesias that extend from the neck and shoulder to the medial aspect of the forearm and hand, ending in the small and ring fingers. Exacerbation of symptoms with overhead activity clouds the distinction between impingement and thoracic outlet syndrome. Perhaps the most important physical sign is the ability to reproduce the patient's symptoms by abducting and laterally rotating the arm at the shoulder while palpating the wrist pulses.[10] Loss of pulse is helpful, but not pathognomonic. Rather, reproduction of symptoms confirms the diagnosis.

The most common cause of misdiagnosis due to intra-articular pathology comes from glenohumeral instability.[6–8,11,12] Instability tends to occur in young athletic individuals with some element of joint laxity who later develop a secondary impingement syndrome. The distinction may be difficult to identify, and reports of many series include cases of instability initially diagnosed and treated as impingement syndrome. Clues to the diagnosis include signs of apprehension with provocative positioning and the presence of joint laxity. To optimize outcome, treatment should be directed at the underlying instability rather than the impingement. Even then, there is a significant challenge in attempting to return this population to preinjury competitive levels.[13–15]

Glenohumeral arthritis and labral tears are also identified sources of misdiagnosis. These are often encountered during the diagnostic arthroscopy portion of the surgical treatment of impingement syndrome. This diagnosis may be complicated by coexisting pathology related to the rotator cuff/impingement problems.[6–8]

Extra-articular pathology as a source of misdiagnosis often includes unrecognized acromioclavicular joint arthritis.[6–8,16–19] This arthritis is a very common cause for recurrent impingement and reoperation in patients who have failed initial decompression surgery. The dilemma stems from the poor correlation between radiographic findings of acromioclavicular joint degeneration

and clinical symptoms. Direct palpation, provocative testing (cross body adduction), and lidocaine injection into the acromioclavicular joint help confirm the diagnosis. Distal clavicle resection has been demonstrated to positively influence outcome after failed initial decompression.

Adhesive capsulitis or primary frozen shoulder may manifest as shoulder pain, but it has an additional component of restricted range of motion. Absolute numbers regarding the limitation of motion are variable, but most agree that there is a significant restriction of glenohumeral motion with both active and passive attempts at range of motion. In contrast, impingement syndrome has a relative full range of motion with pain localized anteriorly during forward flexion.

Many investigators have reported successful results with debridement of a full-thickness cuff tear combined with decompression. But decompression alone in the context of an unrecognized full-thickness cuff tear has been demonstrated to cause continued shoulder pain, which requires reoperation for repair. It is hoped that the incidence of this misdiagnosis will decrease as more surgeons use arthroscopy for decompression with visualization of both the articular and bursal sides of the cuff.

Finally, there are those patients who have undergone surgical management for impingement syndrome whose result may be clouded by factors related to secondary gain or personality. Several reports have documented less reliable results in those patients who had worker's compensation issues still pending.[7,8,20,21] Others have cited psychiatric disorders in the differential for an unsatisfactory outcome.

COMPLICATIONS RELATED TO DECOMPRESSION

DELTOID DETACHMENT
Decompression of the subacromial space has been advocated for rotator cuff disorders since Watson-Jones[22] first described complete acromionectomy in the treatment of supraspinatus tendon lesions. Emphasis centered on increasing

the space available for the rotator cuff to pass beneath the coracoacromial arch. Unfortunately, the early treatment of impingement revolved around a perspective that shoulder abduction was the primary cause of symptoms. As a result, acromionectomy[23–26] and lateral acromionectomy[27] were advocated to increase pain-free abduction. Favorable results were possible, but the potential for complications was realized once the anatomy of impingement syndrome was better articulated and forward flexion was recognized as the primary plane for functional shoulder motion. In addition, the complete removal or lateral resection of the acromion was soon found to increase the risk for disrupting the proximal deltoid attachment. In 1981, Neer and Marberry[28] treated 30 consecutive patients who previously had a radical acromionectomy. All had poor results, including persistent pain, marked weakness of the shoulder, and the inability to raise the arm above the horizontal. They concluded that radical acromionectomy weakened the deltoid both by removing its lever arm and by increasing the postoperative risk of detachment of the deltoid origin. The implications of disrupting the deltoid attachment may be appreciated by understanding that the deltoid muscle, in concert with the rotator cuff, is responsible for generating synchronized and powerful glenohumeral motion. Loss of deltoid muscle integrity results in significant disability. This disability far outweighs the presence of an isolated rotator cuff tear.

Thus, the risk factors shown to correlate highly with deltoid detachment include a history of complete or lateral acromionectomy. In these procedures, a major portion of the fulcrum for the deltoid has been removed. Other conditions noted with this complication include a history of infection/hematoma, postoperative trauma, and/or early aggressive postoperative rehabilitation.[29,30] Detachment typically occurs in the first 6 weeks postoperatively. In general, any situation that involves detaching a portion of the deltoid for exposure increases the risk for subsequent detachment. With modern arthroscopic techniques of decompression in which the deltoid attachment to the acromion is theoretically preserved, this com-plication has not been reported in the literature, but it still could occur if meticulous technique is not followed.

The diagnosis of deltoid detachment depends on identifying the retracted enlargement of the detached deltoid distal to an indentation where the deltoid immediately originates (Fig. 60). Less reliable signs include decreased abduction strength, which often is disabling enough to prevent raising the arm above the horizontal, and/or decreased motion secondary to adherence of the retracted portion of the deltoid to the underlying rotator cuff and humerus. Magnetic resonance imaging (MRI) may confirm the finding (Fig. 61). Conservative treatment of this complication typically demonstrates poor function. In 1994, Groh and associates[29] reviewed the functional results of 33 patients after deltoid detachment. Twenty-two rated their function as poor as determined by activities of daily living, and all reported disability. Other treatment options include attempts at deltoid reattachment, deltoid rotation-plasty, or salvage with glenohumeral arthrodesis. In 1996, Sher and associates[31] evaluated 24 patients who had undergone direct repair or rotational deltoidplasty reconstruction of a detached

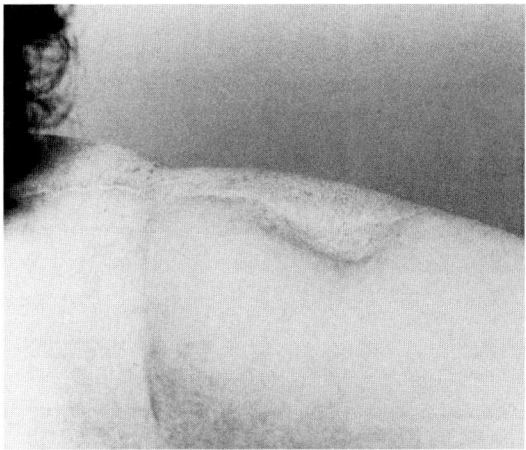

FIGURE 60
Clinical appearance of a postoperative deltoid detachment. (Reproduced with permission from Naranja RJ, Iannotti JP, Gartsman G: Complications of rotator cuff surgery, in Norris TR (ed): *Orthopaedic Knowledge Update: Shoulder and Elbow.* Rosemont, IL, American Academy of Orthopaedic Surgeons, 1997.)

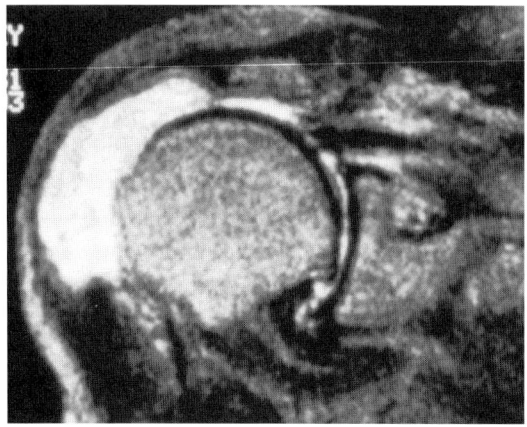

FIGURE 61

T2-weighted coronal magnetic resonance image demonstrating separation of the deltoid from its origin with interposed fluid (high signal). (Reproduced with permission from Naranja RJ, Iannotti JP, Gartsman G: Complications of rotator cuff surgery, in Norris TR (ed): *Orthopaedic Knowledge Update: Shoulder and Elbow.* Rosemont, IL, American Academy of Orthopaedic Surgeons, 1997.)

muscle origin in the setting of prior surgery. They found 67% unsatisfactory results at a mean follow-up of 39 months. Poor outcome with deltoid reconstruction was associated with a prior lateral acromionectomy, involvement of the middle deltoid, a concomitant massive rotator cuff tear, and duration of symptoms greater than 12 months.[31] Both Sher and associates[31] and Groh and associates[29] stress the importance of prevention of this disabling complication, because current nonsurgical and surgical measures to treat deltoid detachment have yielded poor results.

INADEQUATE DECOMPRESSION

Neer[3] has been credited with articulating the anatomy for impingement to include the anterior edge and undersurface of the anterior third of the acromion, the coracoacromial ligament, and in some cases, the acromioclavicular joint. Inadequate decompression is one of the more common reasons for failure after initial surgical intervention for impingement.[3] Analysis of those cases with inadequate decompression reveal that it often results when the decompression technique neglects the anatomy of the impingement

lesion. Consequently, it is not surprising to find that in those cases in which lateral acromionectomy procedures were performed, a high rate of continued impingement occurred because a portion of the impinging anatomy was left behind (Fig. 62). Others have reported attempts simply to divide the coracoacromial ligament.[13,18,32,33] This, too, has resulted in reoperation in several cases.[18] Its role as an isolated procedure in young patients is unclear.

Other cases of inadequate decompression have been related to poor judgment regarding the amount of bone resected with respect to the anterior acromioplasty. In an experimental and computer simulation of anterior acromioplasty, the elimination of impingement was specific to an acromioplasty represented by flattening of the acromion from a location extending from the anterior third to the midline. Anterior acromioplasty alone (flattening of the anterior ridge) resulted in residual impingement, and a flattening of the entire acromion was excessive.[34]

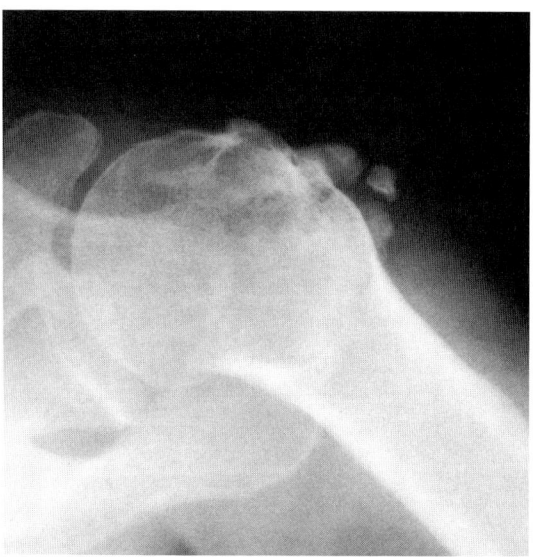

FIGURE 62

Axillary view after lateral acromioplasty in a patient with continued impingement and heterotopic ossification. (Reproduced with permission from Naranja RJ, Iannotti JP, Gartsman G: Complications of rotator cuff surgery, in Norris TR (ed): *Orthopaedic Knowledge Update: Shoulder and Elbow.* Rosemont, IL, American Academy of Orthopaedic Surgeons, 1997.)

In summary, decompression of the subacromial space requires a thorough understanding of those anatomic structures that cause impingement combined with an ability to judge the adequacy of the decompression. Preoperative evaluation includes a clinical examination to determine if acromioclavicular symptoms contribute to the impingement syndrome, as well as appropriate radiographic projections. In a recent study, appropriate radiographic projections for the assessment of acromial morphology have been shown to have good interobserver reliability and correlation with intraoperative measurements of acromial spur size. Specifically, the supraspinatus outlet and 30° caudal tilt have been shown to accurately evaluate acromial morphology, while the axillary view has been less helpful in this regard.[35] Thus, an anteroposterior radiograph in the plane of the scapula, a supraspinatus outlet view, a 30° caudal tilt, and, if confirmed by clinical examination, a 20° cephalic tilt to evaluate the acromioclavicular joint are useful in determining the amount of resection required for an adequate decompression. If an inadequate decompression results, treatment options include conservative therapy with repeat injection and cuff strengthening, or repeat surgical decompression. The results of repeat decompression after failed initial acromioplasty have been relatively good, if persistent outlet narrowing can be demonstrated.

ACROMIAL FRACTURE

Acromial fracture is an infrequent complication related to subacromial decompression. It has been associated with overaggressive decompression of the acromion, as well as overenthusiastic retraction of the acromion during exposure of the rotator cuff. In one series of 74 rotator cuff repairs, one patient (1%) suffered an acromial fracture that required fixation with a screw. Nine months later, deltoid avulsion was noted, the fragment of acromion and the screw were removed, and an attempt was made to resuture the deltoid to the remaining acromion. The long-term outcome was poor.[36,37]

In another series, the results were analyzed of 29 consecutive patients who were treated using an evolving surgical acromioplasty technique. The first group were treated using a surgical technique that required a partial deltoid origin detachment and anterior acromioplasty with an osteotome. The second technique spared the deltoid detachment but again an osteotome was used to perform the acromioplasty. The third technique also spared the deltoid origin, but this time a high speed burr was used to perform the acromioplasty. All complications occurred in the earliest group. One of these patients suffered an acromion fracture.[38]

The difficulty in healing a postoperative or intraoperative acromial fracture is explained by the surgically altered blood supply and the decreased thickness of the acromion, which compromise internal fixation. Arthroscopic subacromial decompression has also resulted in acromial fracture[39] (Fig. 63). Six patients were reported who had poor response to treatment of this complication. Risk factors include osteoporotic bone

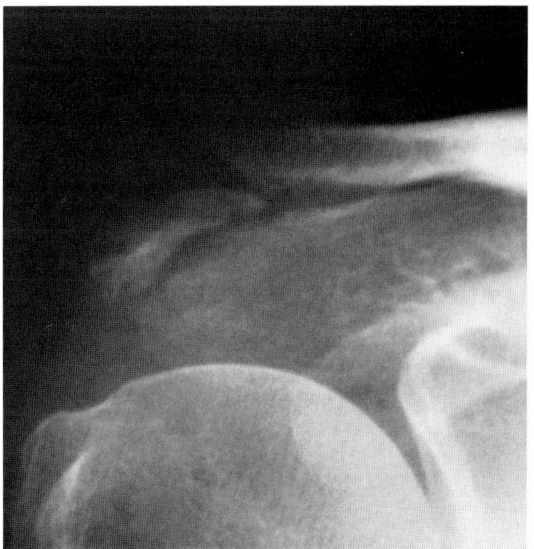

FIGURE 63
Oblique plain radiographic view of the acromion demonstrating the complication of acromial fracture. (Reproduced with permission from Naranja RJ, Iannotti JP, Gartsman G: Complications of rotator cuff surgery, in Norris TR (ed): *Orthopaedic Knowledge Update: Shoulder and Elbow*. Rosemont, IL, American Academy of Orthopaedic Surgeons, 1997.)

and overzealous bone resection.[39] Clearly, the potential for healing complications with an acromial fracture and the apparent failure to consistently respond to attempts at fixation[40] demand careful attention to surgical technique to avoid this infrequent, but serious complication.

HETEROTOPIC OSSIFICATION

Heterotopic ossification as a complication of rotator cuff surgery was reported as early as 1949.[26] Its occurrence at the site of previous acromionectomy caused recurrent impingement symptoms that required reexcision. Subsequent reports of heterotopic ossification have been variable with regard to the development of recurrent symptoms.[23,36,37,41–44] Their incidence has been thought to relate to bone dust remaining after arthroscopic acromioplasty.[43] But others report an association with underlying medical disorders.[42] In one large series of patients who developed heterotopic ossification after distal clavicle excision (Fig. 64) or subacromial decompression, the incidence of heterotopic ossification was 3.2% and was disproportionately seen in patients with a history of chronic pulmonary diseases. No correlation was found between the method of bone resection and incidence of heterotopic ossification. Half of the patients, however, required repeat surgery to remove the ossification. The results of surgery after the formation of heterotopic ossification are related to the size, the site, and the presence of risk factors. Risk factors include a profile of hypertrophic pulmonary osteoarthropathy, active spondylitic arthropathy, and a history of chronic pulmonary disease. It should be understood that bone present on postoperative radiographs does not always represent heterotopic ossification, but rather inadequate initial bone resection. The difference between these two causes of residual bone are best resolved by obtaining postoperative radiographs within the first 4 weeks after surgery.

SUPERIOR GLENOHUMERAL INSTABILITY

The rotator cuff's role in preventing superior migration of the proximal humerus with shoulder abduction and forward flexion is diminished with

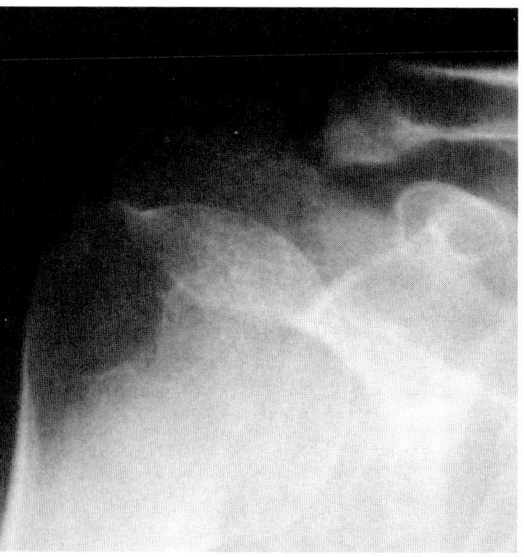

FIGURE 64

Anteroposterior radiograph demonstrating heterotopic ossification at the site of a previous distal clavicle resection. (Reproduced with permission from Naranja RJ, Iannotti JP, Gartsman G: Complications of rotator cuff surgery, in Norris TR (ed): *Orthopaedic Knowledge Update: Shoulder and Elbow*. Rosemont, IL, American Academy of Orthopaedic Surgeons, 1997.)

large full-thickness tears. Later secondary restraint may come from the coracoacromial arch as demonstrated by recent biomechanical studies.[45,46] In one of these studies, 25 cadavers were evaluated using biomechanical testing after sequential interventions of (1) capsular venting, (2) release of the rotator interval capsule and coracoacromial ligament (CAL) connection, (3) release of the CAL at the acromion, and (4) after acromioplasty. Superior translation of the humeral head was increased after CAL release and further after acromioplasty. The authors suggested avoidance of CAL release and acromioplasty in two particular clinical situations: cuff deficiency and patients with high functional demands who poorly tolerate changes in coupled motions (eg, throwing athletes). As a result, careful consideration must be given to reattaching the CAL in these patients. Further removal of the coracoacromial arch complex is deleterious (Fig. 65). Several reports of superior dislocation/subluxation after acromionectomy with an associated large rotator cuff tear have been described.[47,48]

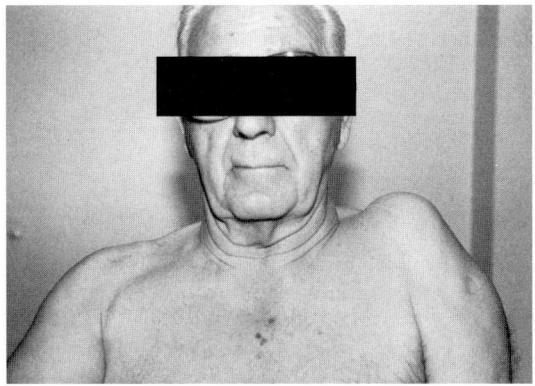

FIGURE 65
Clinical example of superior glenohumeral escape following acromioplasty and coracoacromial ligament resection in a patient with a massive rotator cuff tear. (Reproduced with permission from Naranja RJ, Iannotti JP, Gartsman G: Complications of rotator cuff surgery, in Norris TR (ed): *Orthopaedic Knowledge Update: Shoulder and Elbow.* Rosemont, IL, American Academy of Orthopaedic Surgeons, 1997.)

CLAVICULAR INSTABILITY

In 1988, the results of the Mumford procedure in 23 athletes with a history of grade I or grade II dislocation were analyzed. Ten athletes in the series demonstrated increased horizontal clavicular motion.[49]

In a subsequent evaluation of the results of arthroscopic subacromial decompression in which there also was arthroscopic distal clavicle resection, several patients reported instability of the acromioclavicular joint after vigorous weight lifting within the first postoperative week. The symptoms subsided with several weeks of rest.[50]

In 1993, the complication has been reported of a "dropped shoulder" with the clavicle protruding into the trapezius secondary to distal clavicle resection.[51] The authors identified damage to the superior acromioclavicular capsular ligament as the inciting cause of this instability. The authors further recommended resecting only 1 to 1.5 cm of the distal clavicle with a burr in an attempt to preserve the superior acromioclavicular capsular ligament.[51]

In 1966, Blazar and associates[52] reviewed 17 patients who had a distal clavicle resection and correlated anteroposterior instability based on stress radiographs (Fig. 66) with postoperative pain and functional outcome. They found that increased translation of the distal clavicle after distal clavicle resection was associated with increased postoperative shoulder pain and poor surgical outcome.[52]

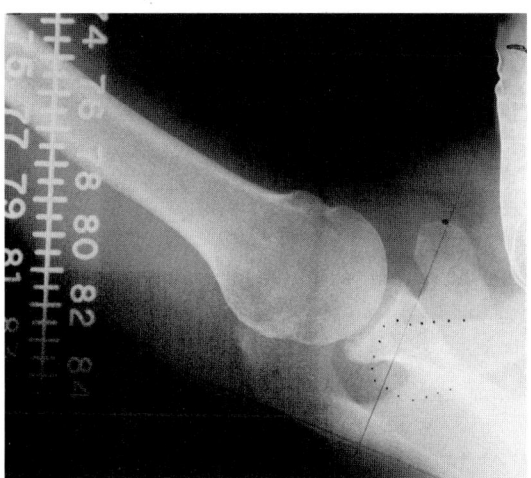
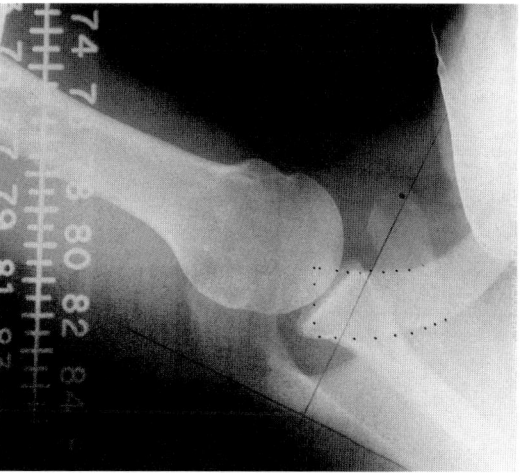

FIGURE 66
Net translation of 7 mm between posterior (**A**) and anterior (**B**) stress testing after distal clavicle resection.

COMPLICATIONS RELATED TO CUFF REPAIR

RECURRENT TEAR

Tears of the rotator cuff have been classified according to their size: small, less than 1 cm; medium, 1 to 3 cm; large, 3 to 5 cm; and massive, greater than 5 cm. Numerous techniques have been described for rotator cuff repair, particularly for large and massive tears. No technique, however, has been immune from a recurrent tear. Recurrence has been attributed to quality of the cuff and size of the tear at the time of repair, inadequate intraoperative mobilization and exposure of the cuff, failure to remove extrinsic impingement processes, poor fixation techniques, posttraumatic falls, or inadequate postoperative protection and spontaneous rupture.[40,53–58]

Recurrent tears from inadequate mobilization and poor exposure of the torn edges of the rotator cuff have been well documented. For example, in 1990, one author reported that at reoperation for failed rotator cuff surgery, thickened hypertrophied bursal tissue was found sutured and closed over a rotator cuff defect. Bursal tissue must be resected if the surgeon cannot gain sufficient exposure to adequately mobilize the underlying cuff.[57] In another series, 25 of 32 patients who underwent postoperative arthrography demonstrated a recurrent or persistent tear. Reasons identified included inadequate exposure and/or mobilization of the cuff as determined by review of the surgical notes.[59]

Gerber and associates[58] have also shown the importance of suture type, suture configuration, and bone quality with regard to the strength of repair. The authors evaluated the mechanical properties of several current techniques of tendon-to-bone suture used in rotator cuff repair. No. 2 nonabsorbable braided polyester sutures best combined ultimate tensile strength and stiffness. A modified Mason-Allen suture technique was superior with regard to tendon grasping. And in cases of osteoporotic bone, the use of a 2-mm thick, plate-like augmentation device improved failure strength over transosseous sutures.

Decompression of the subacromial space has been recommended as a concomitant procedure with rotator cuff repair. In addition to pain relief, this procedure minimizes the chance for a recurrent tear. In 1984, 27 patients were evaluated after initial failed rotator cuff repair. Inadequate decompression of the coracoacromial arch was a major factor for recurrent tears.[54]

The use of synthetic materials, such as carbon, Gore-tex, or Dacron, (W.L. Gore, Flagstaff, AZ) has been attempted to address irreparable massive tears. In 1991, the use of carbon fiber for repair of the rotator cuff in 14 patients was evaluated. One patient was noted to have a recurrent tear by arthrography. Histologic examination 2 years after index repair noted fragmentation of the carbon fibers embedded in a loose connective tissue.[60] Further investigations comparing the mechanical, microangiographic, and histologic results of different synthetic materials in mongrel dogs have confirmed the suggestion that the use of the currently available rotator cuff substitutes cannot be recommended.[61]

Allograft interposition has also been reported to have poor results.[62] The results of freeze-dried allografts in rotator cuff repairs were described in 1988. This series of seven patients in general did not obtain good functional results. One patient underwent reexploration 9 months after surgery, and the allograft was found to be avascular and disrupted.[62]

Other investigators have found that the use of staples to augment rotator cuff repair may be associated with unnecessary complications.[56,63,64] In 1983, a report was published of 63 patients who underwent surgical treatment for a chronic rotator cuff tear. Staples were used to augment the repair in four patients. All required later staple removal, and none had a good result.[64] Similarly, in another review of complications about the glenohumeral joint related to the use of screws and staples, two patients who had a rotator cuff repair with the use of staples experienced staple pull-out and migration into the joint. In one patient, the staple was removed and the cuff was resutured. The other patient refused further treatment.[63]

Postoperatively, patients require cautious rehabilitation, because postoperative falls and inadequate immobilization have been cited as reasons for recurrent tear.[65,66] In one series, four cases of traumatic disruption of rotator cuff repair were described. The mechanism was by a fall in each case.[67,68] In another case of a traumatic recurrent tear, noncompliance with postoperative immobilization resulted in a recurrent tear of a free biceps graft reconstruction. Attempt at a second repair with free biceps graft was unsuccessful.[68]

There also exist reparable tears that have initially been treated with decompression alone, only to later require repair for continued symptoms. This problem has been illustrated in a recent study of arthroscopic subacromial decompression in three different populations.[21] Group 1 had stage II impingement syndrome, group 2 had partial tear of the rotator cuff, and group 3 had a full-thickness rotator cuff tear. Seven patients in group 3 ultimately required an open surgical repair.[69] The result was satisfactory in six of the seven after repair. In another evaluation of the long-term results of 25 patients who underwent arthroscopic subacromial decompression in the treatment of full-thickness rotator cuff tears, eight required later rotator cuff repair.[69] One of the eight experienced an increase in size of his tear from large to massive during this interval.

Clearly, meticulous surgical technique and cautious postoperative rehabilitation will minimize the chance for recurrent tears. But the necessity to completely cover the gap occurring at the site of tear has recently been questioned. Initial recommendations for direct repair advocated obtaining a "watertight closure." This concept, however, was disputed in 1986, when the use of arthrography after surgical repair of a torn rotator cuff in 20 patients at an average of 30 months postoperation was reported.[59] In 18 of 20 patients, contrast medium leaked into the subacromial bursa indicating a defect in the cuff. Results, however, did not correlate with this finding; 17 patients no longer complained of pain, and 15 had a full range of shoulder motion. The authors concluded that a watertight closure is not essential for a good functional result.

Correlation of rotator cuff tear recurrence with results was later analyzed in 1991. One hundred and five surgical repairs of the rotator cuff were evaluated by ultrasonography and correlated with the functional outcome at follow-up.[70] Of those with tears that preoperatively involved the supraspinatus alone, 20% had a recurrent defect. Of those with tears involving more than the supraspinatus, there was a 50% incidence of recurrent defect. Shoulders with an intact cuff at follow-up had better function and had a satisfactory result in 97% of the cases. In contrast, those with a recurrent defect were satisfied in 87% of cases. A high prevalence (55%) of cuff tears was observed by ultrasonography in the opposite shoulder.

In 1991, 97 rotator cuff tears were analyzed postoperatively with the use of ultrasonography.[71] Twenty-nine had complete rupture of the cuff. The authors, however, reported a poor correlation between the clinical and ultrasonographic results. One third of the contralateral rotator cuffs were noted to be abnormal.[71] In contrast, Gazielly and associates[72] found good correlation between outcome and integrity of cuff at follow-up as determined by ultrasound.

Finally, two separate groups of investigators have noted satisfactory results with debridement and decompression alone for massive rotator cuff tears.[73-75] A "functional cuff tear" then becomes the surgical goal for relieving pain and optimizing function.

NEUROLOGIC INJURY

Most open anterior surgical approaches for rotator cuff surgery are performed through a limited deltoid muscle split. Intramuscular axillary nerve injury can result in denervation of the anterior deltoid (Fig. 67). The relationship to the axillary nerve may be understood by recalling its anatomy as it arises from the fifth and sixth cervical roots and forms the posterior cord of the brachial plexus. At the inferior border of the subscapularis, it travels posteriorly under the inferior capsule and joins the posterior humeral circumflex artery to exit the quadrangular space. At this point the axillary nerve divides into anterior and posterior trunks. The posterior trunk gives off branches to the teres minor and posterior deltoid and terminates as the superior lateral cutaneous nerve of the arm. The anterior trunk passes

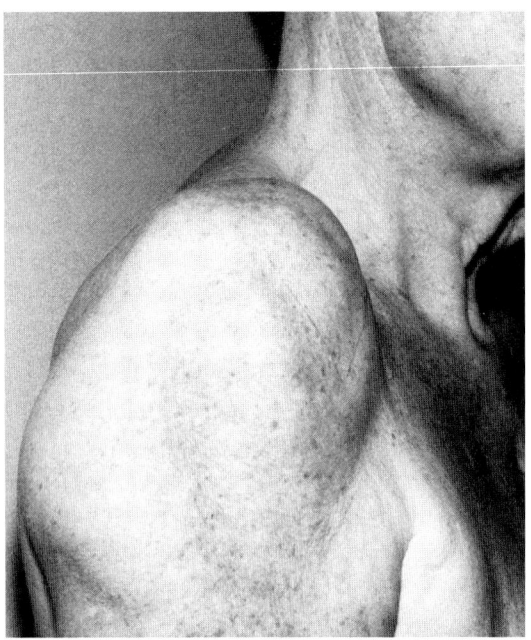

FIGURE 67

Clinical example of significant deltoid atrophy following a rotator cuff repair complicated by deltoid denervation. (Reproduced with permission from Naranja RJ, Iannotti JP, Gartsman G: Complications of rotator cuff surgery, in Norris TR (ed): *Orthopaedic Knowledge Update: Shoulder and Elbow.* Rosemont, IL, American Academy of Orthopaedic Surgeons, 1997.)

anteriorly around the humerus approximately 5 cm distal to the lateral border of the acromion. Tremendous variation in the course and position of the axillary nerve in anatomic studies suggests that this safe zone is only a guideline and careless, overexuberant retraction must be avoided.[76] In 1992, a case of deltoid denervation after acromioplasty and rotator cuff repair was reported. In this case, the extent of deltoid split was 4 cm.[29] Subsequently, in 1994, two cases of axillary nerve palsy after rotator cuff repair for massive tears were described.[77] Fortunately, these recovered within 3 months. The axillary nerve is also at risk in cases of subscapularis repair, and care must be taken in the surgical approach to protect this nerve.[78]

In 1965, the technique of advancement of the supraspinatus muscle in its fossa through a pos-

terior approach in 23 shoulders was described.[79] In no case did electromyography show evidence of nerve injury, but care must be taken in this approach because the suprascapular nerve is in close proximity during this "supraspinatus slide." With respect to a standard anterosuperior approach for cuff repair, Warner and associates,[80] in an anatomic study, demonstrated that the suprascapular neurovascular pedicle only allowed 1 cm of lateral advancement. This represents the actual mobilization of the tendon from its original anatomic position and not the extent of mobilization of retracted tissue. With retracted tissue, the neurovascular pedicle may also be tethered by scar, limiting mobilization even further.[80]

ACROMIAL NONUNION

In 1980, the "supraspinatus slide" of Debeyre was evaluated in 37 patients.[81] The approach is posterosuperior and requires an acromial osteotomy for exposure of the supraspinatus fossa. The authors reported one acromial nonunion requiring a second surgical procedure with screw fixation. Symptoms were subsequently relieved. In 1994, Paulos and associates[82] described an acromion-splitting approach for large and massive rotator cuff tears. In this series of 38 shoulders, there were nine cases (24%) of asymptomatic fibrous union.

COMPLICATIONS RELATED TO POSTOPERATIVE REHABILITATION

FROZEN SHOULDER

The development of a frozen shoulder after rotator cuff surgery may be associated with prolonged immobilization postoperatively, poor patient compliance, and deltoid detachment.[6,17,24,56,67,68,83–85] Treatment options include physical therapy, manipulation under anesthesia, and/or open or arthroscopic release of adhesions.[19,64,68,84,86] Care must be taken during manipulations under anesthesia to avoid excess force and subsequent iatrogenic humeral fracture.

REFLEX SYMPATHETIC DYSTROPHY

Reflex sympathetic dystrophy is a condition characterized by pain, hyperesthesia, vasomotor and sudomotor disturbances, and increased muscular tone, followed by weakness, atrophy, and trophic changes involving the skin, appendages, muscles, bones, and joints. The condition is thought to be a result of noxious stimuli (such as surgery) eliciting an aberrant sympathetic response. Its incidence after rotator cuff surgery is approximately 0 to 2%.[20] Treatment includes pharmacologic therapy, nerve blocks, and if this is unsuccessful, surgical or chemical sympathectomy. Consultation with a pain management service is helpful in addressing this complication.

BICEPS RUPTURE

The long head of the biceps tendon may be involved in the degenerative changes that occur in rotator cuff pathology. As a result, it may become susceptible to rupture after rotator cuff surgery as shown in several reports.[19,24,87] Disability after this injury is minimal, and repair usually is not necessary.

COMPLICATIONS RELATED TO WOUND HEALING

This group of complications includes hematomas, draining sinuses, suture granulomas, superficial infections, and keloids or uncosmetic scars.[3,28,36–38,56,62,64,68,88–96] The risk factors for these complications are, in general, unpredictable. Early recognition and removal of offending tissues typically will result in resolution. More complex is the issue of deep infection.[28,30,67,81,88,97] This situation represents a significant negative impact on the final outcome of surgery. Aggressive debridement and culture-derived parenteral antibiotics are the principle treatments.

REFERENCES

1. Codman EA: Complete rupture of the supraspinatus tendon: Operative treatment with report of two successful cases. *Boston Med Surg J* 1911;164:708–710.

2. Rathbun JB, Macnab I: The microvascular pattern of the rotator cuff. *J Bone Joint Surg* 1970;52B:540–553.

3. Neer CS II: Anterior acromioplasty for the chronic impingement syndrome in the shoulder: A preliminary report. *J Bone Joint Surg* 1972; 54A:41–50.

4. Neer CS II: Impingement lesions. *Clin Orthop* 1983;173:70–77.

5. Sher JS, Urbe JW, Posada A, Murphy BJ, Zlatkin MB: Abnormal findings on magnetic resonance images of asymptomatic shoulders. *J Bone Joint Surg* 1995;77A:10–15.

6. Ogilvie-Harris DJ, Wiley AM, Sattarian J: Failed acromioplasty for impingement syndrome. *J Bone Joint Surg* 1990;72B:1070–1072.

7. Hawkins RJ, Chris AD, Kiefer GN: Failed anterior acromioplasties. *Orthop Trans* 1987;11:233.

8. Hawkins RJ, Chris T, Bokor D, Kiefer G: Failed anterior acromioplasty: A review of 51 cases. *Clin Orthop* 1989;243:106–111.

9. Thorling AJ, Bjerneld H, Hallin G, Hovelius L, Hagg O: Acromioplasty for impingement syndrome. *Acta Orthop Scand* 1985;56:147–148.

10. Leffert RD: Neurological problems, in Rockwood CA Jr, Matsen FA III (eds): *The Shoulder.* Philadelphia, PA, WB Saunders, 1990, vol 2, pp 750–773.

11. Ellman H: Diagnosis and treatment of incomplete rotator cuff tears. *Clin Orthop* 1990;254:64–74.

12. Glousman RE: Instability versus impingement syndrome in the throwing athlete. *Orthop Clin North Am* 1993;24:89–99.

13. Hawkins RJ, Kennedy JC: Impingement syndrome in athletes. *Am J Sports Med* 1980;8:151–158.

14. Tibone JE, Jobe FW, Kerlan RK, et al: Shoulder impingement syndrome in athletes treated by an anterior acromioplasty. *Clin Orthop* 1985; 198:134–140.

15. Tibone JE, Elrod B, Jobe FW, et al: Surgical treatment of tears of the rotator cuff in athletes. *J Bone Joint Surg* 1986;68A:887–891.

16. Altchek DW, Warren RF, Wickiewicz TL, Skyhar MJ, Ortiz G, Schsartz E: Arthroscopic acromioplasty: Technique and results. *J Bone Joint Surg* 1990;72A:1198–1207.

17. Ha'eri GB, Wiley AM: Shoulder impingement syndrome: Results of operative release. *Clin Orthop* 1982;168:128–132.

18. Kessel L, Watson M: The painful arc syndrome: Clinical classification as a guide to management. *J Bone Joint Surg* 1977;59B:166–172.

19. Neviaser TJ, Neviaser RJ, Neviaser JS, Neviaser JS: The four in one arthroplasty for painful arc syndrome. *Clin Orthop* 1982;163:107–112.

20. Hawkins RJ, Brock RM, Abrams JS, Hobeika P: Acromioplasty for impingement with an intact rotator cuff. *J Bone Joint Surg* 1988;70B:795–797.

21. Gartsman GM: Arthroscopic acromioplasty for lesions of the rotator cuff. *J Bone Joint Surg* 1990;72A:169–180.

22. Watson-Jones R (ed): *Fractures and Joint Injuries,* ed 4. Baltimore, MD, Williams & Wilkins, 1962, vol 2.

23. Hammond G: Complete acromionectomy in the treatment of chronic tendinitis of the shoulder: A follow-up of ninety operations on eighty-seven patients. *J Bone Joint Surg* 1971;53A:173–180.

24. Hammond G: Complete acromionectomy in the treatment of chronic tendinitis of the shoulder. *J Bone Joint Surg* 1962;44A:494–504.

25. Hammond G: Abstract: Complete acromionectomy in the treatment of tendinitis of the shoulder. *J Bone Joint Surg* 1961;43A:1260.

26. Armstrong JR: Excision of the acromion in treatment of the supraspinatus syndrome: Report of ninety-five excisions. *J Bone Joint Surg* 1949;31B:436–442.

27. McLaughlin HL: Lesions of the musculotendinous cuff of the shoulder: I. The exposure and treatment of tears with retraction. *J Bone Joint Surg* 1944;26A:31–51.

28. Neer CS II, Marberry TA: On the disadvantages of radical acromionectomy. *J Bone Joint Surg* 1981;63A:416–419.

29. Groh GI, Simoni M, Rolla P, Rockwood CA: Loss of the deltoid after shoulder operations: An operative disaster. *J Shoulder Elbow Surg* 1994;3:243–253.

30. Stuart MJ, Azevedo AJ, Cofield RJ: Anterior acromioplasty for treatment of the shoulder impingement syndrome. *Clin Orthop* 1990;260:195–200.

31. Sher JS, Warner JJP, Groff Y, Wolliams GR Jr, Iannotti JP: Treatment of postoperative deltoid origin disruption. Proceedings of the 12th Open Meeting of the American Shoulder and Elbow Surgeons. Atlanta, GA, February 25, 1996, p 36.

32. Johansson JE, Barrington TW: Coracoacromial ligament division. *Am J Sports Med* 1984;12:138–141.

33. Penny JN, Welsh RP: Shoulder impingement syndromes in athletes and their surgical management. *Am J Sports Med* 1981;9:11–15.

34. Bigliani LU, Colman WW, Kelkar R, et al: The effect of anterior acromioplasty on rotator cuff contact: An experimental and computer simulation. Proceedings of the 11th Open Meeting of the American Shoulder and Elbow Surgeons. Orlando, FL, February 19, 1995, p 32.

35. Kitay GS, Iannotti JP, Williams GR, Haygood T, Kneeland BJ, Berlin J: Roentgenographic assessment of acromial morphologic condition in rotator cuff impingement syndrome. *J Shoulder Elbow Surg* 1995;4:441–448.

36. Wolfgang GL: Surgical repair of tears of the rotator cuff of the shoulder: Factors influencing the results. *J Bone Joint Surg* 1974;56A:14–26.

37. Wolfgang GL: Rupture of the musculotendinous cuff of the shoulder. *Clin Orthop* 1978;134:230–243.

38. McShane RB, Leinberry CF, Fenlin JM Jr: Conservative open anterior acromioplasty. *Clin Orthop* 1987;223:127–144.

39. Matthews LS, Burkhead WZ, Gordon S, Racanelli J, Ruland L: Acromial fracture: A complication of arthroscopic subacromial decompression. *J Shoulder Elbow Surg* 1994;3:256–261.

40. Post M: Complications following anterior acromioplasty and rotator cuff repair, in Bigliani LU (ed): *Complications of Shoulder Surgery.* Baltimore, MD, Williams & Wilkins, 1993, pp 34–43.

41. Berg EE, Ciullo JV, Oglesby JW: Failure of arthroscopic decompression by subacromial heterotopic ossification causing recurrent impingement. *Arthroscopy* 1994;10:158–161.

42. Berg EE, Ciullo JV: Heterotopic ossification after acromioplasty and distal clavicle resection. *J Shoulder Elbow Surg* 1995;4:188–193.

43. Lazarus MD, Chansky HA; Misra S, Williams GR, Iannotti JP: Comparison of open and arthroscopic subacromial decompression. *J Shoulder Elbow Surg* 1994;3:1–11.

44. Petersson CJ: Resection of the lateral end of the clavicle: A 3 to 30-year follow-up. *Acta Orthop Scand* 1983;54:904–907.

45. Moorman CT III, Deng XH, Warren RF, Torzilli PA, Wickiewicz TL: The coracoacromial ligament: Is it the appendix of the shoulder? Proceedings of the 11th Open Meeting of the American Shoulder and Elbow Surgeons. Orlando, FL, February 19, 1995, p 33.

46. Lazarus MD, Yung SW, Sidles JA, Harryman DT II: Anterosuperior humeral displacement: Limitation by the coracoacromial arch. Proceedings of the 11th Open Meeting of the American Shoulder and Elbow Surgeons. Orlando, FL, February 19, 1995, p 18.

47. Michelsson JE, Bakalim G: Resection of the acromion in the treatment of persistent rotator cuff syndrome of the shoulder. *Acta Orthop Scand* 1977;48:607–611.

48. Bakalim G, Pasila M: Surgical treatment of rupture of the rotator cuff tendon. *Acta Orthop Scand* 1975;46:751–757.

49. Cook FF, Tibone JE: The Mumford procedure in athletes: An objective analysis of function. *Am J Sports Med* 1988;16:97–100.

50. Esch JC: Arthroscopic subacromial decompression and postoperative management. *Orthop Clin North Am* 1993;24:161–171.

51. Checchia S, Doneux P: Acromioclavicular resection: Complication in acromioplasty. *J Shoulder Elbow Surg* 1993;2(suppl):S11.

52. Blazar PE, Iannotti JP, Williams GR: Anteroposterior instability of the clavicle after distal clavicle resection. Proceedings of the 12th Open Meeting of the American Shoulder and Elbow Surgeons. Atlanta, GA, February 25, 1996, p 28.

53. Bigliani LU, Cordasco FA, McIlveen SJ, Musso ES: Operative treatment of failed repairs of the rotator cuff. *J Bone Joint Surg* 1992; 74A:1505–1515.

54. DeOrio JK, Cofield RH: Results of a second attempt at surgical repair of a failed initial rotator-cuff repair. *J Bone Joint Surg* 1984; 66A:563–567.

55. Neviaser RJ, Neviaser TJ: Reoperation for failed rotator cuff repair: Analysis of fifty cases. *J Shoulder Elbow Surg* 1992;1:283–286.

56. Post M, Silver R, Singh M: Rotator cuff tear: Diagnosis and treatment. *Clin Orthop* 1983; 173:78–91.

57. Post M: Complications of rotator cuff surgery. *Clin Orthop* 1990;254:97–104.

58. Gerber C, Schneeberger AG, Beck M, Schlegel U: Mechanical strength of repairs of the rotator cuff. *J Bone Joint Surg* 1994;76B:371–380.

59. Calvert PT, Packer NP, Stoker DJ, Bayley JI: Arthrography of the shoulder after operative repair of the torn rotator cuff. *J Bone Joint Surg* 1986;68B:147–150.

60. Visuri T, Kiviluoto O, Eskelin M: Carbon fiber for repair of the rotator cuff: A 4-year follow-up of 14 cases. *Acta Orthop Scand* 1991;62:356–359.

61. Kujat R: Rotator cuff substitutes: An experimental investigation. *J Shoulder Elbow Surg* 1993;2(suppl):S8.

62. Nasca RJ: The use of freeze-dried allografts in the management of global rotator cuff tears. *Clin Orthop* 1988;228:218–226.

63. Zuckerman JD, Matsen FA III: Complications about the glenohumeral joint related to the use of screws and staples. *J Bone Joint Surg* 1984;66A:175–180.

64. Packer NP, Calvert PT, Bayley JI, Kessel L: Operative treatment of chronic ruptures of the rotator cuff of the shoulder. *J Bone Joint Surg* 1983;65B:171–175.

65. Cofield RH, Hoffmeyer P, Lanzer WL: Surgical repair of chronic rotator cuff tears. *Orthop Trans* 1990;14:251–252.

66. Heikel HV: Rupture of the rotator cuff of the shoulder: Experiences of surgical treatment. *Acta Orthop Scand* 1968;39:477–492.

67. Samilson RL, Binder WF: Symptomatic full thickness tears of the rotator cuff: An analysis of 292 shoulders in 276 patients. *Orthop Clin North Am* 1975;6:449–466.

68. Neviaser JS: Ruptures of the rotator cuff of the shoulder: New concepts in the diagnosis and operative treatment of chronic ruptures. *Arch Surg* 1971;102:483–485.

69. Ellman H, Kay SP, Wirth M: Arthroscopic treatment of full-thickness rotator cuff tears: 2- to 7-year follow-up study. *Arthroscopy* 1993;9:195–200.

70. Harryman DT II, Mack LA, Wang KY, Jackins SE, Richardson ML, Matsen FA III: Repairs of the rotator cuff: Correlation of functional results with integrity of the cuff. *J Bone Joint Surg* 1991;73A:982–989.

71. Wulker N, Melzer C, Wirth CJ: Shoulder surgery for rotator cuff tears: Ultrasonographic 3-year follow-up of 97 cases. *Acta Orthop Scand* 1991;62:142–147.

72. Gazielly DF, Gleyze P, Montagnon C: Functional and antomical results after rotator cuff repair. *Clin Orthop* 1994;304:43–53.

73. Rockwood CA Jr, Williams GR Jr, Burkhead WZ Jr: Debridement of degenerative, irreparable lesions of the rotator cuff. *J Bone Joint Surg* 1995;77A:857–866.

74. Burkhart SS, Nottage WM, Ogilvie-Harris DJ, Kohn HS, Pachelli A: Partial repair of irreparable rotator cuff tears. *Arthroscopy* 1994;10:363–370.

75. Burkhart SS: Arthroscopic debridement and decompression for selected rotator cuff tears: Clinical results, pathomechanics, and patient selection based on biomechanical parameters. *Orthop Clin North Am* 1993;24:111–123.

76. Burkhead WZ Jr, Scheinberg RR, Box G: Surgical anatomy of the axillary nerve. *J Shoulder Elbow Surg* 1992;1:31–36.

77. Nobuhara K, Hata Y, Komai M: Surgical procedure and results of repair of massive tears of the rotator cuff. *Clin Orthop* 1994;304:54–59.

78. Gerber C, Hersche O, Farron A: Isolated rupture of the subscapularis tendon. *J Bone Joint Surg* 1996;78A:1015–1023.

79. Debeyre J, Patte D, Elmelik E: Repair of ruptures of the rotator cuff of the shoulder: With a note on advancement of the supraspinatus muscle. *J Bone Joint Surg* 1965;47B:36–42.

80. Warner JP, Kruschell RJ, Masquelet A, Gerber C: Anatomy and relationships of the suprascapular nerve: Anatomical constraints to mobilization of the supraspinatus and infraspinatus muscles in the management of massive rotator cuff tears. *J Bone Joint Surg* 1992;74A:36–45.

81. Ha'eri GB, Wiley AM: "Supraspinatus slide" for rotator cuff repair. *Int Orthop* 1980;4:231–234.

82. Paulos LE, Meislin RJ, Drawbert J: The acromion-splitting approach for large and massive rotator cuff tears. *Am J Sports Med* 1994;22:306–312.

83. Earnshaw P, Desjardins D, Sarkar K, Uhthoff HK: Rotator cuff tears: The role of surgery. *Can J Surg* 1982;25:60–63.

84. Flugstad D, Matsen FA, Larry I, Jackins SE: Failed acromioplasty: Etiology and prevention. *Orthop Trans* 1986;10:229.

85. Levy HJ, Uribe JW, Delaney LG: Arthroscopic assisted rotator cuff repair: Preliminary results. *Arthroscopy* 1990;6:55–60.

86. Snyder SJ, Pachelli AF, Del Pizzo W, Friedman MJ, Ferkel RD, Pattee G: Partial thickness rotator cuff tears: Results of arthroscopic treatment. *Arthroscopy* 1991;7:1–7.

87. Burkhart SS: Arthroscopic treatment of massive rotator cuff tears: Clinical results and biomechanical rationale. *Clin Orthop* 1991;267:45–56.

88. Daluga DJ, Dobozi W: The influence of distal clavicle resection and rotator cuff repair on the effectiveness of anterior acromioplasty. *Clin Orthop* 1989;247:117–123.

89. Neviaser JS, Neviaser RJ, Neviaser TJ: The repair of chronic massive ruptures of the rotator cuff of the shoulder by use of a freeze-dried rotator cuff. *J Bone Joint Surg* 1978;60A:681–684.

90. Cofield RH: Subscapular muscle transposition for repair of chronic rotator cuff tears. *Surg Gynecol Obstet* 1982;154:667–672.

91. Ellman H, Hanker G, Bayer M: Repair of the rotator cuff: End-result study of factors influencing reconstruction. *J Bone Joint Surg* 1986; 68A:1136–1144.

92. Ellman H: Arthroscopic subacromial decompression: Analysis of one- to three-year results. *Arthroscopy* 1987;3:173–181.

93. Ellman H, Kay SP: Arthroscopic subacromial decompression for chronic impingement: Two- to five-year results. *J Bone Joint Surg* 1991;73B:395–398.

94. Speer KP, Lohnes J, Garrett WE Jr: Arthroscopic subacromial decompression: Results in advanced impingement syndrome. *Arthroscopy* 1991;7:291–296.

95. Sahlstrand T: Operations for impingement of the shoulder: Early results in 52 patients. *Acta Orthop Scand* 1989;60:45–48.

96. Post M: Rotator cuff repair with carbon filament: A preliminary report of five cases. *Clin Orthop* 1985;196:154–158.

97. Essman JA, Bell RH, Askew M: Full-thickness rotator cuff tear: An analysis of results. *Clin Orthop* 1991;265:170–177.

INDEX

Distal clavicle resection
  for acromioclavicular arthritis 28
  indications for 30
  results 50–52
  technique 36–39
Disuse osteopenia 21–22, 63

E
Ellman technique 31–32
Epidemiology
  of anterior-superior tears 81
  of posterior-superior tears 59
Etiology, cuff disease
  impingement 5–9
  kinematics 9–12
  multifactorial 4, 12
  of posterior-superior tears 62–64
  tendon degeneration 4–5

F
Fatty degeneration 61, *62*
Fracture, acromial *99*–100
Frozen shoulder 96, 104

G
Glenohumeral arthritis 96
Glenohumeral instability 96, 100–*101*
Gymnasts 27

H
Heterotopic ossification *100*
Horn blower's sign
  in patients with irreparable tears
  77–*78*
  for posterior-superior tears 64, *66*
Hypovascularity, supraspinatus tendon
4–5

I
Imaging
  for acromioclavicular arthritis 27–28
  for anterior-superior tears 84–85
  for impingement syndrome *26*
  for posterior-superior tears 64, 66
Impingement
  and acromial morphology 5–*7*
  and subacromial contact 7–9
  syndrome 25–27
Impingement sign 25, 95

Impingement test 25, 95
Infraspinatus tendon anatomy 1–*3*
Instability
  clavicular 101
  glenohumeral 96, 100–*101*
Irreparable tears
  anterior-superior 89
  defined 76
  latissimus dorsi tendon transfer for
  79–81
  surgical techniques for 76–79

K
Kinematics 9–12
Kissing lesion *34*

L
Langer's lines 67, *68*
Lateral decubitus position
  for arthroscopic acromioplasty 31–33
  for mini-open cuff repair 43
  for open cuff repair 44
Latissimus dorsi tendon transfer
  patient selection for 78–79
  results of *78,* 80–81
  technique 79-80
Lidocaine injection 27
Lift-off test 28, 82–*84*
Ligament anatomy 1–4, 81

M
Magnetic resonance imaging
  for anterior-superior tears 85, *86*
  for posterior-superior tears *62,* 64, 66
Mason-Allen suture repair technique
  for mini-open cuff repair 44, *45*
  for open cuff repair 46
  for optimal holding power *19,* 72–*73*
  preventing recurrent tear with 102
Massive rotator cuff tears
  anterior-superior 81–*90*
  defined 59
  and fatty atrophy of infraspinatus
  muscle 61
  irreparable 76–81, 89
  posterior-superior 62–76
  size of tear and function 60–*61*
Mattress suture technique 19–20, *41*–42
Mechanism of injury

for anterior-superior tears 81
  and posterior-superior tears 62–64
Mini-open rotator cuff repair
  indications for 31
  results 52–53
  technique 43–44
Misdiagnosis
  complications related to 95–96
  and failed arthroscopic acromioplasties 25, 50
Mitek suture anchor 21
Morphology, acromion 5–*7*
Muscle anatomy 1–2, 81
Muscle atrophy 61, *62*

N
Nerve compression, suprascapular 95
Neurologic injury, surgical complication
103–104
Nonabsorbable suture 19, 22, 72, 102
Nonsteroidal anti-inflammatory
medications
  for acromioclavicular arthritis 28
  for impingement syndrome 26
Nonunion, acromial 104
Notchplasty burr 34–36

O
Open rotator cuff repair
  indications for 30–31
  results 53
  technique 44, 46–47
Os acromiale 3
  radiography for 64
Ossification, acromial 3
Osteopenia, disuse 21–22, 63
Osteophytes 6, 26, 27
Outlet view 5, *26,* 64

P
Pants-over-vest sutures 46–*47*
Pectoralis major tendon transfer 89–*90*
Plain radiography. *See* Radiography
Postoperative rehabilitation
  arthroscopic acromioplasty 47
  complications related to 104–105
  latissimus dorsi tendon transfer 80
  massive tear repair 75–76, 89
  rotator cuff repair 47